SMART NUTRITION

How to Feel Great and Live to Be 100

by
Michael J. Grusenmeyer, M.D.

The material in this book is meant for educational purposes only. Readers should consult their individual physicians before implementing the recommendations in this book. Information contained herein should not replace sound medical advice from your personal physician.

To Nicole

From one budding writer to another
Always guard your inner confidence

Contents

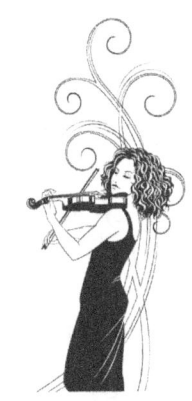

INTRODUCTION

Rocket Fuel

Picture, if you will, the following scenario. Scientists and engineers at NASA have spent years developing and perfecting the Saturn V rocket. Encased in this incredible machine are the latest in scientific advances: the intricate technology and breakthroughs accrued through thousands of hours of research and development by some of the brightest minds in the country. The spaceship that will carry three astronauts to the moon is rolled onto the launch pad at Cape Canaveral, sitting atop the Saturn V. Huge throngs of people crowd the local freeways in the area to watch the launch. Millions of people all over the world sit expectantly in front of their television sets, waiting to enjoy this magnificent spectacle.

And then, incredibly, as part of the final preparation, the ground crew fills the rocket's gas tanks with the lowest grade, cheapest fuel available. The fuel contains impurities that will interfere with proper combustion. After takeoff, the rocket sputters, unable to attain enough power to reach the higher altitudes. The crowd gasps in awe as the rocket surges, misfiring repeatedly and losing power. Reluctantly, NASA aborts the mission. The spaceship falls safely into the sea.

During the subsequent technological analysis of the failed mission, the ground crew is asked why they used such an inferior fuel in such a precisely tuned, finely researched miracle of technology. One crew member replies, "Well, we've always used that." Another crew member, "It was handy." A third says, "We were in a hurry." And a fourth asks, "You mean there's something better we can use?"

Perhaps this scene seems unrealistic, like something out of a bad science fiction movie. Then consider, if you will, the human body. Developed and perfected over millions of years of life on earth, constantly shaped by incredibly powerful forces that demand greater and greater adaptability, the human body is a marvel second to none. The neurological wiring of the human brain alone makes even the most sophisticated computer look like an ancient Chinese abacus.

A Girl in an Orchestra

To understand this, picture, if you will, another scenario. A young woman takes her place as one of a hundred musicians seated in front of a large audience. She and her fellow musicians each hold an instrument that is used to make sounds to please the people who have come to hear their performance. Although only twenty-one, this young woman has practiced violin for fifteen years, often spending eight hours a day learning to play as well as she can. Her eyes read the notes, her mind translates them into movement, and her fingers follow her brain's commands to play thousands of different notes on this instrument. Each note can be played for a varying amount of time, each at a different volume, some softer, some louder, each chosen by the composer from among an almost infinite number of possibilities. Not only can she play by sight but also from memory. Not only can she play this remarkable piece but also hundreds of others, each extremely complex, each entirely different. She is not unique in this ability but shares it with the ninety-nine musicians around her. Even more amazing, they play in such split-second unison that their combined sound, all one hundred instruments, emanates in a fashion that is extremely pleasing to the people who have gathered to hear the musicians perform, to enjoy the music they make.

While she plays, the young woman need not pay attention to the workings of her body. Another lower, more primitive part of her brain will ensure that her heart continues to beat at a healthy pace, that her lungs inhale the proper amount of air to oxygenate her tissues, and that her internal thermostat maintains her body temperature within a narrow physiologic range.

In addition to these cerebral processes, her body functions. All other metabolic processes continue. Her kidneys filter her blood, her intestines digest her dinner, and her liver provides a proper amount of energy to fuel her bodily systems. Even the small injuries she recently sustained to her skin are repaired simultaneously. She constantly makes millions of new cells, especially those with a high turnover rate, such as hair cells, blood cells, and the mucosal cells which line her gastrointestinal tract. Her reproductive system functions so that, should the timing be right, she can begin to develop another remarkable human being. Within each of the billions of cells in her body, a dynamic variety of metabolic processes continues, including cellular energy production, tissue building, and respiration.

Yet she gives no conscious thought to any of these remarkable processes. They are maintained automatically by her subconscious mind while she is attuned to the music. Her goal is to play extremely well, to produce a work of beauty, to please her admirers.

Little wonder, then, that the rocket, marvelous as it is, does not reflect in the least the abilities of our musician. The human body is like nothing ever seen in the fifteen billion-year history of Earth. But the musician, too, like the rocket, like all life in the universe, requires energy to perform. Without it, she withers and dies; with it, she thrives and excels. Energy is the life force for our musician as well as for the NASA rocket. Energy is the fuel of every life and every machine in existence. Without it, there will be no journey for the rocket. Without it, there will be no performance for our young lady. If she is deprived of energy for long enough, she will cease to function, she will no longer survive.

Like the ground crew for the fictitious space ship, the musician has never really paid much attention to the nature of the fuel she supplies to her body. Eating and drinking have usually been an automatic function. During the first eighteen years of her life she ate what was served at home. Since moving out to live independently, she either eats the institutional food offered at the school cafeteria or she frequents the most convenient fast food places that she can find. Occasionally she cooks on her own, but since she often practices music for many hours after attending classes, there is precious little time to devote to choosing nutritious meals.

Few of her colleagues put much thought into their food selection other than considering the taste and cost. Her friends do not consider this unusual, because any fuel will suffice; that is, their bodies will convert it to energy that they can use and that will enable them to perform their daily functions. However, although their bodies can use any food that they consume, much of the fuel contains impurities that can make their systems sputter and fail, just like the rocket.

Yet, if there is one thing that will keep this marvelous musician functioning superbly, now and for another eighty years, it is the food that she consumes. Yes, for another eighty, since she is already twenty years old and she and many of her colleagues may live to the previously rare age of one hundred years or even more. At the turn of the previous century, in the year 1900, average life expectancy in the United States was forty-five years of age. Now, for a newborn of her species and gender born in the year 2000, one century later, the life expectancy is eighty-two years of age - almost double the earlier figure of a century before. Her children may be born in an era with a life expectancy of over a hundred years. But unfortunately, many of the diseases that will take her life and those of her contemporaries could have been averted or delayed with proper choices of lifestyle, including diet. These diseases include all of the top killers, heart attack, stroke, cancer, and diabetes.

The most important factors that determine our longevity are genetics, nutrition, exercise, proper rest, and safe habits. Many people, feeling that they have little control over the first item on this list give up on the other four. Yet, suppose that the body is designed to live between thirty and one hundred years. Those who eat poorly, suffer high stress, use street drugs, smoke cigarettes, abuse alcohol, never exercise, and sleep poorly, will fall on the short end of the range. However, the body is also designed to recover from an incredible amount of abuse, including poor sleep, inadequate nutrition, and the ingestion of toxic substances before it suffers serious long term effects. For example, a young man can destroy half his liver with alcohol but, if he quits drinking, this organ can recover. Similarly, if he stops other poor habits, his body is so designed as to recoup much of its former good health.

Alternatively, let's say that, at a young age, you decide to eat well, handle stress calmly, avoid recreational drugs, refrain from smoking, drink alcohol moderately or not at all, get regular exercise, sleep adequately, and avoid dangerous hobbies, you will fall at the long end of the range of life expectancy, closer to one hundred years. Not only will you live longer, but your body and mind will perform better during your allotted time on the planet. More importantly, *while* you are living those one hundred years, you will feel *so much better* than you would if you didn't follow a healthy lifestyle. So, your choice of lifestyle will determine not only your longevity, but also your level of performance and your level of comfort –in other words, how well you are going to function and feel during those one hundred years. Would you not then want to know how you can improve your performance, just like our musician will ask her teacher how she can render one of Mozart's quartets more beautifully?

The Importance of Nutrition

Nutrition is one of the most important factors under our control that determines longevity. We in the US live in a country where an incredible variety of food is available, from the dismal and abysmal to the delightful and delicious. And to anyone who has traveled to a foreign country, particularly in the third world, one of the nicest conveniences on returning home is the easy accessibility of nutritious, inexpensive food. Several times a day, each of us chooses what fuel to put into our system. In fact, some of us always seem to be eating! Our choice of food plays a significant role in our health, immediately and long into the future.

Perhaps you remember a movie called *Back to the Future*. In it, Christopher Lloyd plays an eccentric scientist who has invented a most unusual car. Lloyd, utilizing Einstein's equation that $E = mc^2$, has designed an engine that can run on literally anything. The engine can convert matter, any matter, to energy. At one point, when he runs out of fuel, Lloyd picks up some garbage from the trash can on the front lawn, tosses it into the fuel tank, and off he goes again.

Many of us treat our bodies in this way. We grab whatever food is available, wherever it's convenient, including junk food from stores attached to gas stations. Many of these foods primarily consist of sugar, salt, bleached flour, and unhealthy oils, plus the ubiquitous artificial colors, flavors, and preservatives. Unfortunately, our body is not like the engine in the movie - it cannot convert any matter into energy without also being affected by the quality of the ingredients. What we eat has a profound impact not only on our energy level, but also on how we feel, perform, sleep, and even on how we age.

Our health correlates with our nutrition. When we eat well, we are healthier, we feel better, we have more energy, our joints are suppler, our bones are stronger, we recover faster after exercise, and we heal more quickly after injury. As we'll see, when we study the diets of different cultures and of healthy individuals, nutrition plays a significant role in longevity and the quality of life. Although other factors, such as heredity, exercise, tobacco, alcohol, sleep, and stress are crucial, few are under our control as much as nutrition. We cannot choose our ancestors or genes, we may be exposed to tobacco smoke in public, we may suffer significant stress from our jobs or relationships, but we can choose our food at each meal, consciously and wisely. As a patient once said to me about her seventy-year old husband, "He's smoked for fifty years, he's been a heavy drinker almost that long, he works extremely hard, but he's always eaten well. I think that's why he's still alive and fairly healthy."

Research has shown that a healthy diet can prevent or modify many diseases, including the following:

> Diabetes mellitus
> Hypertension (high blood pressure)
> Arteriosclerosis (hardening of the arteries)
> Myocardial infarction (heart attack)
> Cerebrovascular accident (stroke)
> Kidney stones
> Gout
> Diverticulosis (tics of the colon)
> Arthritis
> Cataracts (opacities in the lens of the eye)
> Cancer, including lung, breast, colon, pancreas, and
>   prostate cancer

A consistently nutritious diet can help us to feel comfortable, strong, energetic, and agile for a century or even more. With every hearty meal that we consume, we infuse every cell in our body with a healthy nutrient broth that keeps us functioning smoothly. With such a powerful tool at our disposal, we would be wise to take full advantage of its tremendous benefits.

Consider the many senior citizens that you know. Some are undoubtedly active, muscular, spry, and cheerful individuals who appear far less than their age. They stand tall, move easily, are bright and cheerful, and have a willing disposition to take on life's next adventure. They love to travel, try new sports, learn yoga, read the latest best seller, and visit with friends. They are the grandparents who still throw their grandchildren in the air, knowing full well that they can safely guide their return to earth. They long ago learned to care for their health, realizing the tremendous benefits that this practice would pay, better than any amount of interest from money in the bank. They come alive in their retirement. For them, the slogan, "These are the golden years," rings true. Since they have retained the zest and vitality of good health, they continue to enjoy their lives immensely. One can imagine them jumping out of bed in the morning, ready to take on the day.

Now consider other senior citizens whom you know, those who are sedentary, weak, arthritic, and often depressed individuals who appear far older than their chronological age. They walk slowly, shuffling along, bent over. They appear drained of energy. If we were able to look inside them, we would see that their arteries have hardened with plaques, delivering poor blood supply to many vital organs. Their joints have become rigid, ratcheting open like a wrench. Their bones have weakened from poor nutrition and disuse, so that the slightest injury causes a fracture. Their muscles have stiffened so much that getting out of bed becomes an exercise in pain. Every movement becomes a challenge. They clog their doctors' offices with varied complaints, large and small, day in and day out. Their chief topic of conversation is their latest medical visit or their poor health. Some consider themselves lucky to be alive, since many of their contemporaries have already succumbed to preventable illnesses in their fifties and sixties. Most never consider the fact that their lifestyle determines their health and that, even at an advanced age, simple changes can bring about profound differences in their wellbeing.

When I see them in the office and ask, "How are your golden years?" they frequently blurt out, "The golden years? That's a load of bull," or, "Whoever dreamed up that phrase has never been old."

The question is, "Which group will you join?" The choices you make *now* will determine your future.

This book will show you how to join the first group.

John the Maintenance Man

John worked as a maintenance man at a hospital in Detroit, Michigan, where I was an emergency physician. We had known each other for years. A veteran of the armed forces, he received several years' credit toward his retirement from his time in the army.

Unfortunately, John hated his work. He couldn't wait until the day he could retire and he made no secret of it. Every day, at the start of his shift, John would look at his watch, and then look at his coworkers and say, "Eight years, four months, three days, and two hours to go." You could stop John at any time of day and he would tell you the exact amount of time, in years, months, days, hours, even minutes, until he qualified to retire and draw his pension.

Since John and I worked a lot of midnight shifts together, we would often go down to the snack bar to order a late breakfast at three or four in the morning, after the patient flow had slowed to a trickle. John always ordered the same thing - two eggs, hash browns, bacon, and sausage. All of the items were fried. They dripped a pool of grease onto his plate. A couple of times, I encouraged him to eat a better diet, but John felt that his diet would not affect his health. He'd laugh and say, "What's going to happen will happen. I'm not going to worry about it." John also smoked a pack of cigarettes a day. Other than the maintenance work that he did around the hospital, John got no exercise. His greatest exertion was carrying a coil of electrical wire or tightening a pipe.

One day several years ago, I had just started an afternoon shift in the same Emergency Room when my first patient appeared - John, the maintenance man. He was having chest pain. The electrocardiogram showed definite signs of an acute, extensive heart attack. We placed John in a room on a monitor and performed all our usual maneuvers. We took a quick history and performed a brief, focused physical. We started oxygen and placed an intravenous line. We hooked John up to the cardiac monitor. We paged one of the hospital's best cardiologists who fortunately appeared in just a few minutes. John was joking constantly since he knew everyone in the hospital. But underneath it all we knew he was scared to death that he had "bought the farm," as we say in medicine, that this heart attack might kill him.

John was admitted to the hospital. When a cardiac catheterization showed several blocked arteries, as suspected, he underwent emergency open heart surgery. After surgery, John suffered cardiac arrest several times in the coronary care unit. His stay was prolonged for weeks when he went into respiratory failure. He needed an intensive, prolonged course of medical intervention and stabilization. Luckily, after three weeks in the Coronary Care Unit, he recovered sufficiently to be transferred to a regular floor and later to return home.

All this happened fifteen years ago. The good news is that John did survive. But, even better, he decided to make some changes in his lifestyle. He quit smoking, changed his diet, and began to walk. He is now retired. He no longer works a job that he hates so much that he counts the hours until retirement. He loves not working. He is active in the local community and volunteers for many projects. Yet this man almost died at the incredibly young age of thirty-eight because of his health habits. He smoked, ate a diet high in saturated fat, and did not exercise. He continued to work a stressful job that he hated. Most of all, when friends would politely express concern over any of these issues, John would firmly and resolutely put them off.

To look at him, and on paper, John was the picture of health. His weight was within a few pounds of normal and he looked in good shape. His past medical history revealed no major health problems. Underneath the surface, however, his coronary arteries were undergoing major changes that almost killed him. They were narrowing to the point that even the minimal amount of blood necessary to sustain his heart muscle was no longer able to flow through them. When stressed, they rebelled.

Our health is multifactorial - that is, many factors play a role, some more important than others. While physicians and researchers still disagree over which factors are most important, no one debates the value of a good diet. The old saying is true – "You are what you eat." Good nutrition is absolutely essential. One of the best ways, if not the best, to feel strong, live a longer and more dynamic life, maintain your health, and be vital and alive is to eat well consistently, meal after meal, day after day. Often, people ignore or are simply not conscious of unhealthy decisions until they experience a medical emergency. Many people wait until they are seriously ill, even until they have a diagnosis of advanced cancer or sustain a heart attack, to make changes in their lifestyle. The simple truth is that the sooner you examine your daily habits, the better. A great place to start is with your nutrition.

My Goals for You in This Book

My aim in this book is threefold. First, it's my goal to explain clearly and succinctly the basic elements of nutrition without the use of complicated medical terminology. Second, I will provide practical guidelines to make it as easy and fun as possible to eat in a way that will enable your marvelous body to function superbly for one hundred years. I'll include plenty of lists and easy-to-read tables that will enable you to determine the exact nutritional value of the food that you eat. Third, I will discuss the "art of nutrition," ways to make a nutritious diet even more healthy and enjoyable. By learning how to eat mindfully, calmly, and without hurry – the art of nutrition - you can further enhance the life-giving sustenance of your food.

Throughout this book, I will provide many suggestions that are practical, financially reasonable, and time conscious. My goal is to present the material in a lucid and concise manner so that it can be easily remembered.

So, look for information that is:

> Easy to understand
> Easy to remember
> Easy to apply

If my explanations meet these criteria, then you, the intended beneficiary, will be able to use this information to profoundly change how you feel, how healthy you are, and how much energy and vitality you bring to your daily life.

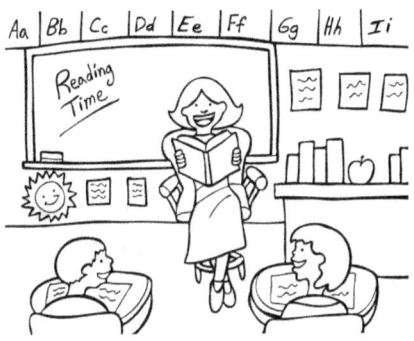

Chapter One – The Basics

Nutrition Terminology

Key Concepts

Let's define a few key concepts. Most of these terms are already familiar to you. The first time that they're used in this book, you'll find them in *italics*, followed by a definition. Don't worry if you can't remember what all these terms mean. They'll make more sense as you progress through the book. My goal in this chapter is to give you a good overview of nutrition. All of these points will be reinforced later and will have increasing significance in your dietary choices.

Nutrition is a function of living animals and plants. In human beings, nutrition refers to the absorption of food for two purposes:

The first purpose of nutrition is to provide fuel or energy.

The second purpose of nutrition is to build up and later break down the cells, which make up the tissue that composes all of our body.

The successive stages of nutrition are:

1.) *Intake* - the ingestion of food into our systems by eating.
2.) *Absorption* - the transfer of nutrients through our intestinal tract, or gut, into the bloodstream.
3.) *Metabolism* - the use of nutrition to provide energy, build new tissue, and break down old tissue. Metabolism is so important that we will discuss it more thoroughly further on.
4.) *Excretion* - the elimination of solid and liquid bodily wastes through the gastrointestinal and urinary tracts in the form of stool and urine, respectively, or, as kids say, pooping and peeing.

Energy

Fuel is any material burned to supply heat or power for any creature or machine: a human being, a pig, a rocket, a furnace, or a car. *Food* is fuel for humans, animals, and even plants. Food and nutrition are not equal terms. Food is the stuff we put into our mouths several times a day. *Nutrition* is a broader term, referring to a series of processes by which an organism assimilates food into itself to provide energy, promote growth, and replace worn out tissues. *Tissue* refers to the structural material or substance of our bodies.

Energy is the ability to utilize fuel, to turn it into work or motion. In human beings, the body uses this fuel to power all bodily processes, including movement, thinking, and growth.

Cars run on gas; we run on calories. In biology, a *calorie* is defined as the amount of heat needed to raise the temperature of one kilogram of water one degree centigrade. Think of a calorie as a small unit of energy. Using the phrase "calories of energy" instead of just "calories," may help to clarify the meaning and eliminate confusion. To simplify, we'll just use the word "calorie." The energy we derive from these calories is the source of power for *everything* that we do.

Energy is the most important concept in nutrition. Our bodies need fuel to work, just like the most intricately crafted rocket or the simplest living being. Without energy, we go nowhere, just like a car that has run out of gas. Without gasoline, even the most luxurious or powerful car becomes just an expensive living room on wheels. Without food, we lose our power to move. Without food, we begin to waste away, as scenes on the evening news of famine in Africa so poignantly demonstrate.

Metabolism

What is metabolism? *Metabolism* refers to the chemical and physical processes continuously occurring in living cells. We think of metabolism as having two phases, a "building up" phase and a "breaking down" phase.

The building up phase is called *anabolism*, where food is converted into the "stuff" that makes up our bodies. This "stuff" is technically called protoplasm. *Protoplasm* is the essential living matter of all animal and plant cells. A *cell* is a small, complex unit of protoplasm enclosed by a membrane. Our body contains hundreds of billions of tiny cells. These cells are so small that, should you scrape your hand, you'll rub off thousands of tiny skin cells.

Each cell contains a *nucleus*, a central oval mass of protoplasm holding most of our genetic material, and a *mitochondrion*, a small power plant that produces energy on a biochemical level. When we eat, we take plant and animal protoplasm and turn it into our own.

Catabolism is the breaking down phase. Catabolism takes old protoplasm and breaks it down into simpler substances. This produces energy and waste products. Humans discard these waste products as stool and urine.

Remember the girl playing the violin? Her body continues to perform all the phases of metabolism, both the building up and the breaking down, while she plays. She builds new cells and breaks down the old into waste products in a continual process from birth to death.

Macro Nutrients

Key Concepts

For human beings, energy comes in three basic food types – carbohydrates, proteins, and fats. These three are also referred to as *macro nutrients* (macro is derived from the Greek *makros* which means long). Thus, a macro nutrient is a long or large nutrient. A *nutrient* is any substance necessary to life and growth. So, macro nutrients refer to carbohydrates, proteins, and fats, the sources of bodily energy. All three macro nutrients can be broken down into a substance called *ATP*, or *adenosine triphosphate*, which is the basic unit of energy in our body that can be used by the cells and tissues. ATP is produced in the mitochondria, the little power houses in our cells. Since this is a handbook of nutrition, we'll leave the elaborate discussion of the formation of ATP to the biochemistry textbooks.

Some nutritionists define macronutrients as any substance that our body needs in large amounts daily. Using this definition, there are actually five macronutrients:

1.) Carbohydrates
2.) Proteins
3.) Fats
4.) Water
5.) Large minerals

The first three macronutrients, carbohydrates, proteins, and fats, are the only sources of energy for the human body. Energy from these nutrients can be stored until the body needs it.

Carbohydrates are stored as *glycogen* in the liver and muscles. Glycogen is the principle carbohydrate reserve of the body. Glycogen is converted to glucose and other monosaccharides for the body's use. A *monosaccharide* is a carbohydrate that cannot be broken down into a simpler sugar. *Glucose* is the medical term for the common sugar in the bloodstream. A *disaccharide* is the condensation product of two monosaccharides.

Fats are converted to *fatty acids*, the building blocks of fats.

Proteins are broken down into their building blocks, *amino acids*, which can be processed as fats or carbohydrates. Amino acids can also build the body's own specific types of proteins.

Most solid foods are composed primarily of one energy source - carbohydrate, fat, or protein. This provides an easy way to categorize food for its nutritional value. Most foods also contain small amounts of the other two nutrients.

The last two macronutrients, water and large minerals, contain no energy but perform other vital bodily functions. *Water* is a clear, odorless, tasteless, and transparent liquid, which becomes solid at 32° Fahrenheit (0° Centigrade) and becomes a gas at 212° Fahrenheit (100° Centigrade). Water is so ubiquitous that it is found in all animal and vegetable tissues and in nearly all other substances. Water is the chief component of all bodily fluids and secretions, including blood, urine, saliva, tears, gastric juices, and cerebrospinal fluid - the liquid that bathes our brain and spinal cord. Our blood is 50 – 60% water. Scientists believe that water is so essential to life that even extraterrestrial life cannot exist without it.

The fifth group of macronutrients, large minerals, may not be familiar to most readers. Large minerals include the following:

1.) Sodium
2.) Chloride
3.) Potassium
4.) Calcium
5.) Phosphorous
6.) Magnesium

Electrolytes are large minerals that maintain the normal acid-base balance in the body. The first three large minerals named above, sodium, chloride, and potassium, are electrolytes. Common table salt, NaCl, contains one atom each of sodium and chloride. Potassium is plentiful in fruits and vegetables.

We'll learn much more about these five groups throughout this book.

Carbohydrates

Carbohydrates are polymers of hexoses. A *polymer* is simply a chain of repeated basic units. The basic unit in this chain, the *hexose*, contains six carbon units in its structure and follows the formula of six carbon atoms, twelve hydrogen atoms, and six oxygen atoms, or $C_6H_{12}O_6$. Unless you're a chemistry student, you won't need to remember this.

Saccharides, or simple sugars, are small carbohydrates with names that usually end in –ose. If you look up saccharide in the medical dictionary, you will find that "sugar" and "carbohydrate" are listed in the definition. Three examples of saccharides are *glucose* (blood sugar), *fructose* (fruit sugar), and *lactose* (milk sugar).

Glucose is the main product of carbohydrate digestion and the main sugar circulating in the body. Your doctor may check your glucose level, especially if you have a personal or family history of diabetes or if you are suffering from "low energy." The normal range is between 50 and 120 milligrams. If your level is below 50, you are *hypoglycemic*, meaning you have low blood sugar. If your level is above 120 while you are fasting or above 160 after eating, then you are *hyperglycemic*, meaning you have high blood sugar. Amazingly, every drop of blood in your body reflects this value. For this reason, diabetics can test their blood glucose level anywhere on their body and obtain the same results. Glucose is the only energy source that the brain can use. If your blood glucose drops too low, you may become drowsy or even comatose.

Starches are large carbohydrates. The large carbohydrates in our food are mostly starches, like grains. A *grain* is defined as the small, hard seed of a cereal plant, such as barley, rye, oats, wheat, or corn. *Glycogen* is the principal carbohydrate reserve in the body, found mostly in the liver and muscles, and is readily converted to glucose.

Vegetables and fruits are mostly carbohydrate. A *vegetable* is defined as the edible part of an herbaceous plant. These edible parts include the root (carrot), tuber (potato), stem (celery), leaf (lettuce), and seed (peas). A *tuber* is a short and thick underground stem.

A *fruit* is the sweet, fleshy, edible part of the plant structure. Botanists describe a fruit as the ovary of a flowering plant.

Occasionally, there is overlap and confusion. Corn is considered a grain and a vegetable, as is the potato. The tomato is considered a vegetable but is technically a fruit. These distinctions aren't important. Fruits, vegetables, and grains are mostly carbohydrate and are derived from the plant kingdom. Fish, red meat, and poultry are part of the animal kingdom. We'll learn more about the animal products further on.

The *glycemic index* is a term coined by researchers to measure how rapidly a particular food increases your blood sugar. Several diet book authors have placed tremendous weight on the importance of this term. However, this research is still in its infancy. A particular food does not have a set glycemic index. Rather, the glycemic index depends on how the food is ripened, processed, stored, and cooked. The index is not a miracle answer to the question of how to control blood sugar. For now, you can safely ignore the glycemic index. You'll find it more valuable to understand concepts such as vitamins, minerals, fiber, and calories (energy).

So, to summarize: Carbohydrates consist of repeating chains of hexoses. *Sugars*, like lactose in milk, are small carbohydrates. *Starches*, like grains, are large carbohydrates. Fruits, vegetables, and grains are mostly carbohydrate.

Proteins

Proteins are also made up of repeated chains. The building blocks are called *amino acids*. Unlike carbohydrates, amino acids contain nitrogen. There are twenty amino acids in protein. Nine are *essential* amino acids, meaning that we must consume these amino acids because our body can't make them. There are eleven *non-essential* amino acids. Our body can make non-essential amino acids even if they aren't in our diet. So, a good diet contains all the essential amino acids that our body can't make.

Proteins occur in all animal and vegetable matter. It's difficult to find a food without some protein in it. The highest concentration of protein is in foods containing flesh, or muscular tissue, from the meat of animals or fish. Humans and other carnivores consume an incredible array of previously living tissue containing mostly protein. Let's define some of these food sources.

Meat is the edible flesh of animals used as food. Some nutritionists distinguish red meat from poultry. *Red meat* includes beef, pork, and lamb. *Poultry* includes domesticated fowl such as chicken and turkey. In a sense, poultry is meat that can fly.

Vertebrate animals have a spinal column or backbone; *invertebrate* animals don't. *Fish* are defined as cold-blooded vertebrates with fins, gills, and a cartilage skeleton. A *shellfish* is an aquatic animal that has an exoskeleton or shell, including crustaceans and mollusks. *Crustaceans* are invertebrate animals with a segmented body. They live in the water and breathe through gills. Edible species include shrimp, crab, and lobster. *Mollusks* are marine invertebrates with a soft body and a protective shell. Edible species include oysters, clams, snails, squid, mussels, and octopus. *Seafood* is a more inclusive term that includes fish and shellfish that are edible by humans. Meat and seafood are mostly protein. However, as we'll see, some red meat contains large amounts of saturated fat.

Protein isn't very efficient for the processes of metabolism (tissue growth, maintenance, repair, and breakdown). The body will break down protein if the preferred sources of metabolism – carbohydrates and fats – aren't available. For this reason, a high protein diet isn't as healthy as a *balanced* diet. Also, people with kidney disease have trouble filtering the breakdown products of protein and so are often placed on a low protein diet.

Fats

Fats are oily compounds primarily found in the bodies of animals.

However, fats are also found in much smaller amounts in plants, usually in seeds. Fats, like carbohydrates and proteins, also contain chains of compounds. These compounds are called, logically enough, *fatty acids.*

To understand the various types of fats, we can briefly study their chemistry. Fatty acids have an even number of carbon atoms in a straight chain. The number of hydrogen atoms attached to each carbon atom is what differentiates these fatty acids. Usually, a carbon atom carries two hydrogen atoms. Picture a chain of adults linked together with a rope and following each other. Each adult holds two children, one with each hand. Every adult represents a carbon atom; each child represents a hydrogen atom.

When making choices about foods that contain fat, what's crucial to know is how saturated that fat is – in other words, how many hydrogen atoms each carbon carries.

In a *saturated fat,* all carbon atoms carry the maximum number of hydrogen atoms, like a line of adults, each holding two children, one in each hand.

In a *monounsaturated fat,* one carbon atom is not saturated at all, so monounsaturated fat contains two hydrogen atoms less than saturated fat. Think of a line of adults, each holding two children except for one adult, who holds none.

In a *polyunsaturated fat,* two or more carbon atoms are not saturated, so polyunsaturated fat contains four or more hydrogen atoms less than saturated fat. Think of a line of adults, two or more of who are holding no children. All essential fatty acids are polyunsaturated fatty acids. (However, not all polyunsaturated fatty acids are essential).

Trans fatty acids are created when manufacturers hydrogenate vegetable oil. They add hydrogen to a polyunsaturated vegetable oil, making some of the unsaturated fat more saturated. Doing this creates a more solid consistency and adds to the life of the product, allowing it to sit on the shelf longer without spoiling. However, trans fatty acids act like saturated fats in the body. What's convenient for the manufacturer is often unhealthy for the body.

The important thing to remember is that saturated fat clogs the arteries much more quickly than any other food. Clogged arteries are a leading cause of heart attacks and strokes. Saturated fat has also been linked to certain types of cancer, such as breast cancer, colon cancer, and possibly prostate cancer.

Remember that, for virtually every topic that we discuss in this book, research is ongoing. In medicine, it is difficult to prove a causal (cause and effect) relationship between a food and a disease. So, we often say "associated with" or "linked to" instead of "caused by." Recently, saturated fat has been associated with the formation of cataracts in the lens of the human eye.

Saturated fat tends to clog up a lot of bodily structures, just like pouring lard down your sink would cause your plumbing to clog up rather quickly. Isn't it amazing that human beings who wouldn't pour grease down their kitchen sink for fear of clogging the plumbing in the house will eat the same material and clog up their own arteries?

The foods that contain most fat are meat and oils. *Oil* is a greasy, combustible substance. *Edible oils* are derived from animal or vegetable sources. *Mineral oil* is derived from petroleum and is used as a laxative, not as a food.

Oils are liquid at room temperature. They're not soluble in water and contain no water. All oils contain a mixture of saturated, mono-unsaturated, and polyunsaturated fatty acids. Each oil is characterized by the predominant type of fatty acids present in the oil. However, the ratios of these fatty acids vary wildly in different oils, as we'll discover later.

The body needs *essential fatty acids* to function properly. Essential fatty acids, like essential amino acids, must be provided in the diet, since our body cannot make them. Omega-6 fatty acids include linoleic and arachidonic acids. Omega-3 fatty acids include alpha-linolenic, eicosapentaenoic, and docosahexaenoic acids. Vegetable oils provide linoleic and linolenic fatty acid. Marine fish oil provides eicosapentaenoic and docosahexaenoic acids (EPA and DHA). You'll find these abbreviations on the ingredient list of fish oil capsules. Research shows that these two fish oils may stabilize heart cells, thereby suppressing irregular heart beats and decreasing sudden death. This tremendous benefit remains subject to ongoing research.

Don't let these tongue twisters confuse you. With names this complex, you can see why these fatty acids are often abbreviated to Omega-3 and Omega-6.

Generally, Omega-3 fatty acids are found in fish. However, walnuts have a significant amount of Omega-3. Some oils, notably flaxseed oil, contain a significant amount of Omega-3, followed by canola and soy. The other oils contain much smaller amounts.

Omega-6 fatty acids are mostly found in plants, especially in oils derived from plants. Remember that both Omega-3 and Omega-6 are polyunsaturated fatty acids.

The following table may clarify the picture.

Polyunsaturated Fatty Acids	
Omega-3	**Source**
Eicosapentanoic (EPA)	Fish
Docosahexaenoic (DHA)	Fish; supplements from algae
Alpha-linolenic	Flaxseed, canola, soy oils, soybeans, walnuts
Omega-6	**Source**
Linoleic	Oils derived from plants

A *triglyceride* is the main type of fat found in body tissues and in foods and is composed of three fat molecules (hence "tri" meaning three) attached to one molecule of the alcohol glycerol. Triglycerides that are liquid at room temperature are called *oils*; those that are solid at room temperature are called *fats*.

Oils usually contain much more unsaturated fatty acids than do fats. As we'll see, this is one reason why fish is considered healthier than meat. Fish from cold seas, such as the Arctic and Antarctic, generally contains less saturated triglycerides than fish from warm seas. Otherwise, their bodies would become stiff at the colder temperatures they encounter, since saturated fats harden quicker in cold temperatures.

Cholesterol, found in the cell walls of all animals, is the most abundant steroid in animal tissue. Cholesterol is not technically a fat but a steroid. The difference is that the carbon atoms of *steroids* are in a ring structure.

However, high levels of cholesterol have damaging effects on blood vessel walls similar to high levels of saturated fats. Since their behavior is similar, physicians often talk about cholesterol and triglycerides in the same sentence. Cholesterol is transported in the bloodstream in different forms. *HDL cholesterol* (high density lipoprotein) protects against cardiovascular diseases like heart attack and stroke; *LDL cholesterol* (low density lipoprotein) increases the chances of these diseases. An easy way to remember the difference is to think "H for healthy, L for lousy."

Fats carry a bad reputation since they contain so many calories. But fats aren't the villains they're made out to be. You may ask, "What's good about fats?" First, they provide a lot of energy. While carbohydrates and proteins provide four calories of energy per gram, fats provide nine calories of energy per gram - more than twice as much. Fats are a great source of energy. If your body craves calories, as in a period of malnutrition or high demand, then a fried, fatty food provides them, much more than a protein or carbohydrate food. This comes at a cost of the health complications mentioned earlier. However, as we will see, there are healthy fats and unhealthy fats.

"What's a gram?" you ask. Perhaps you remember this from high school chemistry class where you used the metric system, now common in most of the world except the United States. A *gram* is a tiny amount of weight. It takes twenty eight grams to make an ounce. So, a gram is 1/28th of an ounce, or about the weight of a paper clip.

Later, when we look at food tables to determine vitamin and mineral content, we'll usually use "100 grams of edible portion" as the basic amount of food. So, if you've done the math, you know that 100 grams is about three and one-half ounces.

Fats not only provide more energy per gram than carbohydrates or protein, but are essential to life. Fatty acids are vital components of membranes. Every cell in our body is surrounded by a *membrane*, a thin structure that has the primary purpose of protecting the cell by controlling what enters and what leaves. Animals fed a fat free diet *do not thrive*. They develop lesions on the kidneys and skin, become infertile, and fail to grow. So, a fat-free diet is not a healthy diet.

Some people have the notion that the lower the fat, the healthier the diet. However, we need to obtain enough calories from our food to supply all our energy needs. Diets that are low in fat are often high in carbohydrates, especially starches and refined sugars. But eating too many carbohydrates can raise the body's level of triglycerides, which has been implicated in heart attack and stroke. Recent popular diets, such as the Atkins diet, have implied that the lower the carbohydrate content of your food, the healthier the diet. Unfortunately, this is misleading. As we'll see, many carbohydrates, such as vegetables, fruits, and whole grains, are extremely healthy.

What's the answer? So far, research shows that the best diet is a *balanced* diet, including all three macro nutrients - carbohydrate, protein, and fat. Although researchers still argue over the exact numbers, the current recommendation is a diet roughly composed of 50% carbohydrate, 30% protein, and 20% fat. Less than half the fat should be saturated, or no more than 10% of your total caloric intake.

Some researchers, flipping the protein and fat percentages, now advise a diet composed of 50% carbohydrate, 20% protein, and 30% fat, with virtually all of the fat unsaturated. We won't quibble about this difference. Remember that diets high in <u>saturated</u> fat have been implicated in coronary artery disease and in various cancers. Also, since fats provide more calories per gram than protein or carbohydrate, high fat diets are high in calories, exactly what an obese patient doesn't need.

Not only is the concept of a balanced diet one of the most important we can learn, but in each of the three macro nutrient food groups - carbohydrates, protein, and fat - there are healthy choices and unhealthy choices.

Micro Nutrients

Food not only contains energy, or fuel, but also other nutrients, sometimes called *micro nutrients*, since they are smaller in size and weight than the macro nutrients. Micro is from the Greek *mikros*, meaning small. *Micro nutrients* are vitamins and trace minerals. These are essential to bodily processes such as balancing the acid-base balance of the blood or as catalysts for metabolic processes. A *catalyst* is a substance that accelerates a chemical reaction but isn't changed or consumed in it. You may want to think of them as "movers and shakers." Most of these metabolic processes take place on the cellular level and are beyond the scope of this book. You can find information on the nutrients that act as catalysts for specific metabolic processes in the helpful table called "Vitamins, Minerals, and Essential Fatty Acids" at the end of this chapter.

Vitamins

A *vitamin* is an organic substance made by plants with the help of sunlight or bacteria. Vitamins are catalysts that facilitate chemical reactions in the body but aren't primary ingredients in them. For example, *thiamin* (vitamin B_1) is a catalyst in the conversion of carbohydrate to usable energy. *Riboflavin* (vitamin B_2) is a catalyst for chemical reactions in the body that release energy from proteins. *Folate* is a cofactor in cell division and growth. Many vitamins perform more than one function.

Vitamins are *organic* substances, that is, they all contain carbon in their molecular structure. Vitamins must be obtained from food or supplements since, with rare exceptions, we cannot make them in our bodies. Vitamins contain no calories (energy), so they can't act as substitutes for the macro nutrients, carbohydrate, protein, and fat, to provide fuel. A person who attempts to diet on vitamins and water alone will have no source of energy other than burning body stores.

Patients who suffer from anorexia nervosa eat so little that they obtain inadequate energy for even their most basic metabolic processes. If the disease is severe enough, these patients eventually begin to break down the protein in their bodies, including that in muscles such as the heart. This condition eventually leads to death due to ventricular fibrillation, in which the heart beats so rapidly and ineffectively that no blood is pumped to the tissues. Vitamins provide no source of energy or calories for these patients.

Vitamins present in food are called *natural* vitamins; those made in a laboratory are called *synthetic* vitamins. Sometimes the name changes slightly depending on the source. The B vitamin *folate* is found in food; *folic acid* is synthetic.

The important thing to remember is that if you lack a particular vitamin some process of metabolism can't proceed properly. *Hypovitaminosis*, or the lack of a vitamin in the diet, causes a disease called a *deficiency state*, since you are deficient in this vitamin. For example, lack of Vitamin C causes *scurvy*. Sailors used to get this on long sea voyages before they began taking lime juice on ship with them. Limes and other citrus fruits are rich in Vitamin C. The most obvious effect of scurvy was bleeding gums, which the sailors inevitably got after just a few weeks at sea.

Similarly, a lack of Vitamin D causes *rickets*. When a patient has rickets, the bones don't form well. Children in impoverished countries have weak, poorly formed, brittle bones. This is most easily seen in the ribs, which become knobby, forming the "rachitic rosary," a series of knobs in the ribs in the shape of a large rosary. We rarely see scurvy or rickets in advanced civilizations.

Generally, vitamins are classified into two groups, fat-soluble and water-soluble.

The fat-soluble vitamins are:

Vitamin A
Vitamin D
Vitamin E
Vitamin K

Water-soluble vitamins include Vitamin C and the eight B vitamins. Thus, the water-soluble vitamins are:

Vitamin C	Pyridoxine (B_6)
Thiamine (B_1)	Cyanocobolamin (B_{12})
Riboflavin (B_2)	Folate
Niacin (B_3)	Biotin (formerly called
Pantothenic acid (B_5)	Vitamin H)

The names of the B vitamins don't make sense. For example, even though there are only eight B vitamins, cobalamin is also called B_{12}. While most of the B vitamins have a number afterward, some don't, such as Folic Acid. Just remember that they're water-soluble.

The fact that our body can't make vitamins, coupled with our constant energy needs, are the two reasons why nature makes hunger such a powerful craving (so much so that some of us seem to do nothing but eat). We must frequently replenish our bodily stores of fuel and vitamins or become sick and perish. Once the body stores of a particular vitamin run out, we become deficient. The exact amount of time we can store each vitamin varies. The fat-soluble vitamins, A, D, E, and K, and one B-Vitamin, B_{12}, generally last much longer than the water soluble vitamins. Thus, we need to replace our stores of the water-soluble vitamins more often than the fat-soluble ones and B_{12}. Patients who suffer from deficiency states are most often seen in countries whose population suffers from malnutrition.

Minerals

Minerals, basic elements that have their origin in the soil, are also essential to the physiology of the body. Animals obtain minerals from eating plants, other animals, or animal products (milk, eggs). In contrast to vitamins, minerals are *inorganic* materials, that is, they contain no carbon in their structure. Minerals often function to build body structures. For example, *iron* is a component of hemoglobin, the part of the red blood cell that carries oxygen in the bloodstream. *Calcium* and *phosphorous,* two of the large minerals mentioned before in the section on macronutrients, make up the basic structure of bones and teeth.

Trace minerals occur in extremely small concentrations in the body. What is an "extremely small concentration"? Trace minerals weigh less than 0.005% of body weight. Nevertheless, they are also essential for health. Large minerals were listed previously under macro nutrients. Trace minerals include the following:

Iron	Selenium
Iodine	Manganese
Fluorine	Molybdenum
Zinc	Copper
Chromium	

Humans apparently don't need some trace minerals that may be necessary in an animal diet. These minerals include the following:

Aluminum	Nickel
Arsenic	Silicon
Boron	Vanadium
Cobalt	

There is ongoing research about the number and type of minerals our body really uses. They remain more mysterious than vitamins.

A table will help us understand just what nutrients are vital to the body.

A Table of Essential Nutrients

Let's take a look at all the nutrients that we need for a healthy, strong body. There is no need to memorize this material. You may want to glance at the source of the different vitamins and minerals, in other words, the foods where they're found. Also, note the effects on the body if we are in a deficiency state, that is, if we don't receive enough of these nutrients. This table is reprinted with the kind permission of Merck[1].

[1]Reprinted with permission. Excerpt from The Merck Manual of Diagnosis and Therapy, Edition 17, pp. 4 – 9, edited by Mark H. Beers and Robert Berkow. Copyright 1999 by Merck & Co., Inc., Whitehouse Station, NJ.

Vitamins, Minerals, and Essential Fatty Acids

Nutrient	Principal Sources	Functions	Effects of Deficiency and Toxicity
Vitamin A (retinol)	As preformed vitamin: fish liver oils, liver, egg yolk, butter, cream, Vitamin A-fortified margarine. As proVitamin Carotenoids: dark green leafy vegetables, yellow fruits, red palm oil.	Photoreceptor mechanism of retina, integrity of epithelia, lysosome stability, glycoprotein synthesis.	**Deficiency**: Night blindness, perifollicular hyperkeratosis, xerophthalmia, keratomalacia, increased morbidity and mortality in young children. **Toxicity**: Headache, peeling of skin, hepatosplenomegaly, bone thickening.
Vitamin D (cholecalciferol, ergocalciferol)	Ultraviolet irradiation of the skin (main source); fortified milk (main dietary source), fish liver oils, butter, egg yolk, liver.	Calcium and phosphorus absorption; resorption, mineralization, and maturation of bone; tubular reabsorption of calcium.	**Deficiency**: Rickets (sometimes with tetany), osteomalacia. **Toxicity**: Anorexia, renal failure, metastatic calcification.
Vitamin E group (alpha-tocopherol and other tocopherols)	Vegetable oil, wheat germ, leafy vegetables, egg yolk, margarine, legumes.	Intracellular antioxidant, scavenger of free radicals in biologic membranes.	**Deficiency**: RBC hemolysis, neurologic damage, creatinuria, ceroid deposition in muscle. **Toxicity**: Interference with enzymes.

Vitamins, Minerals, and Essential Fatty Acids (continued)

Nutrient	Principal Sources	Functions	Effects of Deficiency and Toxicity
Vitamin K group (phylloquinone and menaquinones)	Leafy vegetables, pork, liver, vegetable oils, intestinal flora after newborn period.	Formation of prothrombin, other coagulation factors, and bone proteins.	**Deficiency**: Hemorrhage from deficiency of prothrombin and other factors, osteoporosis.
Essential fatty acids (linoleic, linolenic, arachidonic, eicosapentaenoic, and docosahexaenoic acids)	Vegetable seed oils (corn, sunflower, safflower), margarines, marine fish oils.	Precursors of prostaglandins, leukotrienes, prostacyclins, thromboxanes, and hydroxy fatty acids; membrane structure.	**Deficiency**: Growth cessation, dermatosis, water loss, peripheral neuropathy.
Thiamine (vitamin B1)	Dried yeast, whole grains, meat (especially pork, liver), enriched cereal products, nuts legumes, potatoes.	Carbohydrate metabolism, central and peripheral nerve cell function, myocardial function.	**Deficiency**: Infantile or adult beriberi (peripheral neuropathy, heart failure, Wernicke-Korsakoff syndrome), dependency states.
Riboflavin (vitamin B2)	Milk, cheese, liver, meat, eggs, enriched cereal products.	Many aspects of energy and protein metabolism, integrity of mucous membranes	**Deficiency**: Cheilosis, angular stomatitis, corneal vascularization, amblyopia, sebaceous dermatosis.
Niacin (nicotinic acid, niacinamide)	Dried yeast, liver, meat, fish, legumes, whole-grain enriched cereal products.	Oxidation-reduction reactions, carbohydrate metabolism.	**Deficiency**: Pellagra (dermatosis, glossitis, GI and CNS dysfunction)
Vitamin B6 group (pyridoxine, pyridoxal, pyridoxamine)	Dried yeast, liver, organ meats, whole-grain cereals, fish, legumes.	Many aspects of nitrogen metabolism (e.g., transaminations, porphyrin and heme synthesis, tryptophan conversion to niacin), linoleic acid metabolism.	**Deficiency**: Convulsions in infancy, anemia, neuropathy, seborrhea-like skin lesions, dependency states. **Toxicity**: Peripheral neuropathy.

Vitamins, Minerals, and Essential Fatty Acids (continued)

Nutrient	Principal Sources	Functions	Effects of Deficiency and Toxicity
Folic acid	Fresh green leafy vegetables, fruits, organ meats, liver, dried yeast.	Maturation of RBCs, synthesis of purines, pyrimidines, and methionine.	**Deficiency**: Pancytopenia, megaloblastosis (especially in pregnancy, infancy, malabsorption), dependency states.
Vitamin B12 (cobalamins)	Liver, meats (especially beef, pork, organ meats), eggs, milk and milk products.	Maturation of RBCs, neural function, DNA synthesis related to folate coenzymes, methionine synthesis.	**Deficiency**: Pernicious anemia, fish tape worm and vegan megaloblastic anemia, combined system disease, dependency states.
Biotin	Liver, kidney, egg yolk, yeast, cauliflower, nuts, legumes.	Carboxylation and decarboxylation of oxaloacetic acid; amino acid and fatty acid metabolism.	**Deficiency**: Dermatitis, glossitis, metabolic acidosis, dependency states.
Vitamin C (ascorbic acid)	Citrus fruits, tomatoes, potatoes, cabbage, green peppers.	Essential to osteoid tissue, collagen formation, vascular function, tissue respiration, and wound healing.	**Deficiency**: Scurvy (hemorrhages, loose teeth, gingivitis, bone disease)
Sodium	Wide distribution – beef, pork, sardines, cheese, green olives, corn bread, potato chips, sauerkraut.	Acid-bas balance, osmotic pressure, blood pH, muscle contractility, nerve transmission, sodium pumps.	**Deficiency**: Hyponatremia, confusion, coma. **Toxicity**: Hypernatremia, confusion, coma.
Chloride	Wide distribution – mainly animal products but some vegetables; similar to sodium.	Acid-base balance, osmotic pressure, blood pH, kidney function.	**Deficiency**: Hypochloremic, hypokalemic alkalosis; failure to thrive in infants. **Toxicity**: increase in extracellular volume, hypertension.

Vitamins, Minerals, and Essential Fatty Acids (continued)

Nutrient	Principal Sources	Functions	Effects of Deficiency and Toxicity
Potassium	Wide distribution – whole and skim milk, bananas, prunes, raisins, meats.	Muscle activity, nerve transmission, intracellular acid-base balance and water retention.	**Deficiency**: Hypokalemia, paralysis, cardiac disturbances **Toxicity**: Hyperkalemia, paralysis, and cardiac disturbances.
Calcium	Milk and milk products, meat, fish, eggs, cereal products, beans, fruits, vegetables.	Bone and tooth formation, blood coagulation, neuromuscular irritability, muscle contractility, myocardial conduction.	**Deficiency**: Hypocalcemia and tetany, neuromuscular hyperexcitability. **Toxicity**: Hypercalcemia, GI atony, renal failure, psychosis.
Phosphorus	Milk, cheese, meat, poultry, fish, cereals, nuts legumes.	Bone and tooth formation, acid-base balance, component of nucleic acids, energy production.	**Deficiency**: Hypophosphatemia, irritability, weakness, blood cell disorders, GI tract and renal dysfunction. **Toxicity**: Hyperphosphatemia in renal failure.
Magnesium	Green leaves, nuts cereal, grains, seafood.	Bone and tooth formation, nerve conduction, muscle contraction, enzyme activation.	**Deficiency**: Hypomagnesemia, neuromuscular irritability. **Toxicity**: Hypermagnesemia, hypotension, respiratory failure, cardiac disturbances.
Iron	Wide distribution (except dairy products) – soybean flour, beef, kidney, liver, beans, clams, peaches. Heme iron in meat well absorbed (10-30%); nonheme iron in vegetables poorly absorbed (1-10%)	Hemoglobin and myoglobin formation, cytochrome enzymes, iron-sulfur proteins.	Deficiency: Anemia, dysphagia, koilonychia, enteropathy, decreased work performance, impaired learning ability. Toxicity: Hemochromatosis, cirrhosis, diabetes mellitus, skin pigmentation.

Vitamins, Minerals, and Essential Fatty Acids (continued)

Nutrient	Principal Sources	Functions	Effects of Deficiency and Toxicity
Iodine	Seafood, iodized salt, eggs, dairy products, drinking water in varying amounts.	Thyroxine (T4) and triiodothyronine (T3) formation, energy control mechanisms, differentiation of fetus.	**Deficiency**: Simple (colloid, endemic) goiter, cretinism, deaf-mutism, impaired fetal growth and brain development. **Toxicity**: Hyperthyroidism or myxedema.
Fluorine	Seafood, vegetables, grains, tea, coffee, fluoridated water (sodium fluoride 1.0-2.0 ppm).	Bone and tooth formation.	**Deficiency**: Predisposition to dental caries, osteoporosis. **Toxicity**: Fluorosis, mottling and pitting of permanent teeth, exostoses of spine.
Zinc	Meat, liver, eggs, oysters, peanuts, whole grains; bioavailability variable in plant sources.	Component of enzymes; skin integrity, wound healing, growth.	**Deficiency**: Growth retardation, hypogonadism, hypogeusia Cirrhosis and acrodermatitis enteropathica cause zinc deficiency (secondary).
Copper	Organ meats, oysters, nuts, dried legumes, whole-grain cereals.	Enzyme component hemopoiesis, bone formation.	**Deficiency**: Anemia in malnourished children, Menkes' (kinky-hair) syndrome **Toxicity**: Hepatolenticular degeneration, some biliary cirrhosis.
Chromium	Brewer's yeast, liver, processed meats, whole-grain cereals, spices.	Promotion of glucose tolerance.	**Deficiency**: Impaired glucose tolerance in malnourished children, some diabetics, and some elderly persons.

Vitamins, Minerals, and Essential Fatty Acids (continued)

Nutrient	Principal Sources	Functions	Effects of Deficiency and Toxicity
Selenium	Wide distribution – meats and other animal products; plant content varying with soil concentration.	Component of glutathione peroxidase and thyroid hormone iodinase.	**Deficiency**: Cardiomypathy of Keshan disease, muscle weakness **Toxicity**: Loss of hair and nails, nausea, dermatitis, polyneuritis.
Manganese	Whole-grain cereals, green leafy vegetables, nuts, tea.	Component of manganese-specific enzymes; glycosyltransferases, phosphoenolpyruvate carboxykinase, manganese-superoxide dismutase.	**Primary deficiency:** Questionable **Secondary deficiency** due to hydralazine: Arthralgia, neuralgia, hepatosplenomegaly
Molybdenum	Milk, beans, breads, cereals.	Component of co-enzyme for sulfite oxidase, xanthine dehydrogenase, and one aldehyde oxidase.	**Deficiency**: Tachycardia, headache, nausea, disorientation (sulfite intoxication syndrome).

The table lists twenty-eight nutrients that we need to obtain from our food supply – twenty-seven vitamins and minerals plus essential fatty acids. Our body can store only a handful of them for long periods. We need to obtain the other nutrients on a regular basis.

You may note that every single nutrient has a *deficiency state*. If we fail to consume a sufficient amount of the nutrient, we will suffer physical symptoms and disease. Some nutrients also have a *toxicity state*, which we may suffer if we consume too much. Many of these toxicity states are associated with medical problems, such as kidney failure, in which an excessive amount builds up in the body due to the inability of the kidneys to filter them properly. However, there are documented cases of toxicity in otherwise healthy patients who consume excessive amounts of certain vitamins in their food. The important point is that we don't want to ingest excessive amounts of those nutrients that can cause toxicity. More is not better than enough.

Some foods come close to being "nature's perfect foods," in that they contain many different nutrients. Look at the small but much-maligned egg, for example. An egg contains vitamins A, D, and E, riboflavin, B$_{12}$, biotin, calcium, iodine, and zinc. As you can see from the table, most of these are in the yolk. Whole grains contain Vitamin E, thiamin, niacin, vitamin B6, calcium, fluorine, zinc, copper, chromium, manganese, and molybdenum. However, no single food contains all the nutrients we need.

The key is this - you don't have to know the vitamin and mineral content of every food or even every food group. You only need to know the general principles. Two of these you've already learned. First, consume adequate food as a source of fuel to supply all of your body's energy needs. Second, obtain all of the essential nutrients, the vitamins, minerals, and fatty acids that your body needs for the processes of metabolism. In this book, I'll show you how to make sure and ingest all the important macro nutrients and micro nutrients necessary to provide everything necessary for a healthy body.

Fiber

Fiber is the indigestible part of the carbohydrates in plants. This carbohydrate contains bonds, which cannot be broken down by our digestive enzymes. Therefore, fiber contains no calories available to the body for conversion to energy.

There are two types of fiber.

Soluble fiber can dissolve in water. It's found in oats, barley, beans, and most fruits, including citrus fruits, apples, and strawberries. Soluble fiber may offer protection against coronary artery disease and diabetes. Oats are frequently cited for their ability to lower cholesterol.

Insoluble fiber can't dissolve in water but rather absorbs water. Insoluble fiber helps to soften and bulk up the stool, thus serving as a natural laxative by aiding the rapid transit of stool through the intestinal system and helping to prevent hemorrhoids and constipation. Since fiber increases the speed of transit of solid bodily waste through the intestines, potentially irritating chemicals, like the nitrites found in processed meats, spend less time in contact with the intestinal wall.

Patients who eat a high-fiber diet may be less susceptible to colon cancer. Insoluble fiber is found in bran, whole wheat, barley, brown rice, beans, and some vegetables.

As opposed to saturated fat, which tends to create problems in the body by clogging the arteries, fiber tends to provide opposing benefits. A diet high in fiber helps to lower the blood level of saturated fats and cholesterol. This helps to keep the arteries open, decreasing your chances of serious cardiovascular diseases such as heart attack and stroke. Diabetics in particular will find it more valuable and easier to look for foods that are high in fiber rather than those that are low on the glycemic index.

Free Radicals, Antioxidants, and Phytochemicals

As you may have noticed, the nutrition vocabulary changes frequently which confuses many people. Since our metabolism has changed little over the last several thousand years, we won't be reinventing the wheel. The basic principles remain unaltered. However, there are several recent terms used frequently in the literature that you will want to know in order to understand the latest articles.

A *free radical* is a molecular fragment, or group of atoms, that can be produced by natural biological processes inside the body or can be introduced from the outside. Free radicals can damage our DNA (our genetic code), cells, and proteins by altering their chemical structure. Some external sources of free radicals are tobacco smoke, toxins, and pollutants. Also, molecules of fats that are heated above 500° Fahrenheit during cooking may break apart into free radicals.

Antioxidants inhibit oxidation. *Oxidation* is a chemical reaction promoted by oxygen. In this case, oxidation allows free radicals to form potentially carcinogenic compounds in the body. A *carcinogenic* compound is one that can cause cancer. In other words, antioxidants are the good guys that prevent free radicals from forming. Antioxidants are found mostly in colorful fruits and vegetables and in some grains.

Phytochemicals are chemicals found in plants. (Phyto is from the Greek *phuto* meaning plant.) Many of these "plant chemicals" are pigments that give fruits and vegetables their color. Researchers have already identified almost two thousand plant pigments and continue to discover even more, so it's not important or feasible to remember them. They are widely believed to have tremendous health benefits.

A Summary of the Chapter

Food is the fuel that provides energy for our bodies and minds. We consume this fuel and convert it into calories to sustain our body's processes (metabolism), both the building up (anabolism) and the breaking down (catabolism). Our food consists of macro nutrients (fats, carbohydrates, proteins, water, and large minerals) and micro nutrients (vitamins and trace minerals). They function to provide energy for our cells and catalysts for the body's chemical processes. Fiber is an indigestible part of the carbohydrate found in plants and contains no calories.

Free radicals are nasty compounds that are produced by our body or come from outside sources, such as tobacco smoke, toxins, pollutants, and fats cooked at high heat. They are formed by a chemical reaction called oxidation. Free radicals potentially wreak havoc on our body by altering the chemical structure of our cells, protein, and DNA and can cause cancer. Antioxidants, the good guys that prevent free radicals from forming, are mostly found in colorful fruits and vegetables and in some grains.

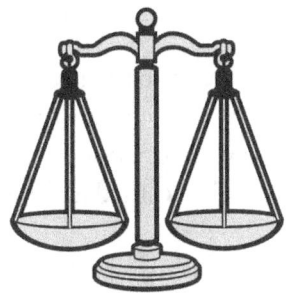

Chapter Two - Determine Your Needs

How Much Food Should You Eat?

You now know to consume adequate food as a source of fuel to supply all of your body's energy needs. While this sounds simple in principle, you may ask, "How much food should I eat?" How much is enough? How many calories do I need? The answer can be simple or complex. The following story may illustrate the difference.

During my first two years of medical school, known as the basic science years, we had approximately thirty hours of lectures per week for forty weeks of the year. Most of the lectures lasted one hour. Before the age of Power Point presentations, virtually every professor taught using slides, which where projected onto a large screen at the front of the room. Some professors brought as many as three carousels of slides, each holding fifty slides. In other words, they projected one hundred fifty slides during a one hour lecture! In addition, some slides held huge amounts of information – graphs, charts, lists, formulas, and so on, often in fine print. The amount of information presented on even one slide could be overwhelming. The class would invariably groan on seeing one of these slides, not knowing what was essential to learn or, more crucial to our success, what would be on the exam.

I remember that one of our professors used lots of slides. That was Dr. Frank McDonald, a nephrologist (kidney specialist). Some of the most complicated equations in medical school refer to the filtering abilities of the kidney. When Frank projected a slide filled with an overwhelming amount of information, he would call these "Oh, my God!" slides. He always chuckled when he drew the inevitable groan from the medical students after projecting one of these monstrosities on the screen. He then went on to reassure us, saying, "Relax. Don't worry. All I want you to know is <u>this</u>." He told us the key elements to remember, those few bits of information from that complex slide that were most important. We all breathed a sigh of relief as our fears of failing the exam faded.

Dr. Frank grew tall in our estimation for his comforting comments. My hope is that you find this book similarly comforting.

So, here's the easy way to know how much to eat. Determine your desirable weight. Now, eat enough calories to stay within five percent of this weight. Simple, huh?

Patients who stay close to their desirable weight live longer. Heavy people die young. Obesity is one of the leading lifestyle factors contributing to early death, second only to smoking. The risk of early death increases with the degree of obesity. That is, the heavier you are, the earlier your death. For most patients, an increase in weight results in a decrease in both the length and quality of life.

Obesity has been linked to a great number of medical problems, including heart disease, diabetes, cancer, high blood pressure, high cholesterol, and even arthritis and gout. The earlier the onset of obesity, the greater the decrease in life expectancy. One simple but vital way to live longer is to stay within five percent of your ideal body weight.

As an aside, some physiologists argue that it is better to be five percent *over* your ideal weight rather than five percent *under*. They reason that, should you encounter a period of your life where you can't eat well, such as during a prolonged illness or after an operation requiring a lengthy recovery, your body has reserves of energy. The same is true during a period of increased demand on the body, such as strenuous exercise, intense labor, or recovery from a significant injury, for example, burns or broken bones.

How do you determine your desirable weight? There's the hard way and the easy way. The hard way involves performing complex calculations that consider multiple factors including the amount of fat as a percentage of body weight, the ratio of the circumference of the waist to the hip, and so on. As Dr. Frank would say, relax. We won't be considering any of these formulas. The easy way is to look at insurance tables. These consider obvious factors such as your gender, height, and frame size (small, medium, or large). You probably already know your gender. If not, then you need more help than I can offer in this book! Your height is easily measured, if not already known. Just knowing these two factors will put you on the correct horizontal line of the graph.

You can obtain a rough estimation of your frame size in the following manner: encircle one wrist with the thumb and middle finger of the opposite hand. If your thumb and middle finger overlap considerably, you have a small frame. If they just meet, you have a medium frame. If there is a large gap between the two digits, you have a large frame. Since some people have long fingers while others have stubby fingers, this method is not completely accurate. Just looking at your wrist can give you a good idea of your frame size.

Let's look at two tables, one for men and one for women. Choose the correct table for your gender and then look at the left hand column for your height. Read across the table to find the desirable weight for your approximate frame size. How did you do?

A Table of Desirable Weights

Height & Weight Table for Women

Height Feet Inches	Small Frame	Medium Frame	Large Frame
4' 10"	102-111	109-121	118-131
4' 11"	103-113	111-123	120-134
5' 0"	104-115	113-126	122-137
5' 1"	106-118	115-129	125-140
5' 2"	108-121	118-132	128-143
5' 3"	111-124	121-135	131-147
5' 4"	114-127	124-138	134-151
5' 5"	117-130	127-141	137-155
5' 6"	120-133	130-144	140-159
5' 7"	123-136	133-147	143-163
5' 8"	126-139	136-150	146-167
5' 9"	129-142	139-153	149-170
5' 10"	132-145	142-156	152-173
5' 11"	135-148	145-159	155-176
6' 0"	138-151	148-162	158-179
Weights at ages 25-59 based on lowest mortality. Weight in pounds according to frame (in indoor clothing weighing 3 lbs.; shoes with 1" heels)			

Height & Weight Table for Men

Height Feet Inches	Small Frame	Medium Frame	Large Frame
5' 2"	128-134	131-141	138-150
5' 3"	130-136	133-143	140-153
5" 4"	132-138	135-145	142-156
5' 5"	134-140	137-148	144-160
5' 6"	136-142	139-151	146-164
5' 7"	138-145	142-154	149-168
5' 8"	140-148	145-157	152-172
5' 9"	142-151	148-160	155-176
5' 10"	144-154	151-163	158-180
5' 11"	146-157	154-166	161-184
6' 0"	149-160	157-170	164-188
6' 1"	152-164	160-174	168-192
6' 2"	155-168	164-178	172-197
6' 3"	158-172	167-182	176-202
6' 4"	162-176	171-187	181-207
Weights at ages 25-59 based on lowest mortality. Weight in pounds according to frame (in indoor clothing weighing 5 lbs.; shoes with 1" heels)			

These tables, issued by the Metropolitan Life Insurance Company[1], have been used for years. Insurance companies have used these statistics from thousands of their customers to determine which characteristics determine health and longevity. The weights they use are those which predict the longest lives.

Recently these tables have fallen out of favor. Met Life was reluctant to release them to me for this book. Critics argue that the insurance company tables are unrealistic and that the weights given are too low.

Although the insurance companies no longer emphasize these tables, new research is underway using "caloric restriction." Researchers previously discovered that primates such as monkeys, who share ninety-five percent of the human gene pool, live far longer when they eat a severe calorie-restricted diet than when they can eat to their satisfaction. New research is underway using human subjects who consume a diet so restricted in calories that it's considered a "near starvation" diet. Preliminary results show findings in people similar to those in primates. So, perhaps the insurance tables are not out of date.

[1] Reprinted with permission of the Metropolitan Life Insurance Company, 1 Met Life Plaza, New York. Copyright 1996 and 1999. This information is not intended to be a substitute for professional medical advice and should not be regarded as an endorsement or approval of any product or service.

You may wish to keep an eye on the research. However, in my experience with thousands of patients, this Spartan diet is too strict for the vast majority of people who do not wish to tolerate a near starvation regimen. However, the point to remember is that people who maintain a healthy body weight live longer.

Keep in mind that the tables provide general guidelines. Not everyone fits conveniently into these categories. After finding your ideal weight, see if it's reasonable for you. You may need to factor in your activity level. In medicine, we use three terms to describe the activity level, going from least to most active. These are sedentary, active, and very active. Now that some athletes train for thirty to forty hours per week in preparation for marathon or triathlon events, we also use the term "extremely active."

Even then, we find variation. A ballerina will want to have a lower body weight than a lumberjack. Both fall in the very active group; what they do for a living is very different. However, no matter what you do for a living, it is not good to fall too far off the tables. Ballerinas, like actresses, often try to fit an ideal image held in the public eye; lumberjacks, even though they are incredibly fit due to the extremely high level of physical activity they undertake each day, don't need to worry about presenting a graceful public image. Dancers are known for being dangerously thin, even anorexic; lumberjacks may eat the wrong kinds of foods, carry around a spare tire, and have high cholesterol levels.

We need to remember several points from the tables. First, extremes at either end are dangerous. Obese people often die in their fifties; patients with anorexia nervosa often die in their teens and twenties. Second, regardless of your gender, height, frame size, or activity level, you are healthiest staying within five percent of your ideal body weight. Whether you sit on your butt most of the day or run one hundred miles per week, seek to maintain a healthy weight. If you do, you are getting adequate calories to fuel your activity, no matter how active. Give yourself the best chance at longevity.

Some fitness experts argue that it is better to be "fat and fit" than to be "skinny and unfit." My advice is that you skip these articles. The studies are uniformly negative about the effects of obesity. Fat kills. The best combination is to maintain a healthy weight _and_ to be fit.

Should this be difficult for you, see your physician for a complete exam. Address any medical problems. Then, a referral to a nutritional counselor may help. If you are unsure whom to see, simply ask your physician or call the local hospital. The visit may save your life.

The Breslow Seven

Insurance companies are not alone in their findings. Dr. Lester Breslow, Dean of the UCLA School of Public Health, studied the charts of thousands of patients in the 1950s. He came up with his famous list of seven health habits that he found in those patients that lived the longest. They have since become known as the Breslow Seven. A recent medical journal article showed Dr. Breslow, now in his nineties, taking a walk with his wife. Thousands of studies have been conducted since his pioneering work but none have improved on the seven habits.

They are as follows:

1.) Get regular exercise.
2.) Eat regular meals.
3.) Eat breakfast every day.
4.) Maintain a normal weight.
5.) Don't smoke.
6.) Use alcohol moderately, if at all.
7.) Get seven to eight hours of sleep a night.

Interestingly, three of the seven habits, numbers two, three, and four, involve diet. Those who maintain a desirable body weight live longer, healthier lives. Those annoying middle-aged or elderly people who brag that they weigh the same amount as they did in college have reason to be proud (as long as they weighed a desirable amount in college).

Recently, I treated a sixty-eight year old patient who complained of a loss of energy. He weighed 240 pounds as opposed to his weight of 180 in high school. At six feet tall, he was well over the desirable weight found in the tables, even for a man with a large frame. As we began the workup for his problem, I noted that, compared to his senior year of high school, he was now fifty years older and carrying the equivalent of a sixty pound back pack everywhere he went.

Should he choose to get rid of the back pack, he might well notice a lighter spring in his step and a reservoir of increased energy. While he couldn't subtract fifty years from his age, he could certainly increase his vitality by losing considerable weight.

Eating breakfast is a simple way to improve your health. I am constantly amazed at the number of patients who tell me they eat no breakfast at all or eat an unhealthy "meal," such as coffee and a donut. As many as one half of all adults and one quarter of children eat nothing before going to work or school. Although it seems counter-intuitive, people who skip breakfast weigh more than those who eat breakfast. After fasting all night and through the morning hours, hunger pangs set in. Most people grab what's handy at work, often a donut, a bagel with cream cheese, or anything from the vending machines, like cookies, candy, potato chips, or soda. But the high fat, sugar, salt, and caffeine content of these foods isn't what the body needs. Eating a nutritious breakfast at home is far healthier. As we'll see in a subsequent chapter, whole grain cereal, fruit, and low-fat dairy products make a better meal.

Mind you, it's normal to eat. Hunger signals a need for energy. Indeed, hunger is an early sign of starvation. Skipping breakfast deprives the brain of glucose, its only energy source. When we go for long periods without eating, we score poorly in tests of memory and concentration. Children who don't eat breakfast perform poorly on exams.

If you fast from dinner the previous night and skip breakfast the next morning, then your body is using its stored energy for fifteen to twenty hours. We constantly use energy, even while asleep, and our body must burn reserves during that time. We must replenish these stores. Obese patients in particular need to eat regular healthy meals.

So, eat a healthy breakfast. Eat regular meals. Maintain a normal weight. If you do, you've already achieved three of the Breslow Seven.

Food as a Drug

Every primary care physician has experienced the following scenario: an obese middle-aged patient comes to the office. She has diabetes and her blood sugar has been perilously high. Typically, the patient doesn't follow a diet, gets no exercise, and is resistant to taking insulin. She states, "I hate needles so I don't want insulin shots. I don't like to exercise. I have a hard time losing weight. Doctor, just give me the pill."

There are pills to treat diabetes. But, as an internist friend of mine loves to say, "The first three treatments for diabetes are, "Number one, diet, number two diet, and number three, diet." In my opinion, number four is exercise. Number five is medication.

You may not be obese or even diabetic. But, on any given day, virtually all the patients seen in the doctor's office complain of feelings of fatigue, being tired every day, or of having no energy. If the doctor told you that there is a powerful medicine that give you more energy, build strong bones, open and cleanse blood vessels, make you feel younger, and let you live longer, would you not demand to know what it is?

There is such a powerful drug. We take this drug three times a day in large quantities. Some of us ingest it five to ten times daily.

This drug is called food.

If you begin to think of your nutrition as the most powerful drug you can put into your mouth, meal after meal, snack after snack, day after day, you will be on the path to creating a healthy body. There is no pill that comes close to having this powerful effect on your body. No medicine is even in the same league. You don't need steroids, amphetamines, caffeine, performance enhancers, memory aids, energy boosters, or exotic herbs. For the most part, you don't need supplements.

You need to eat well. This book will tell you how. Meanwhile, begin to think of food as a powerful a drug designed by nature to energize you and bring you to the peak of health. Use it wisely.

Recommended Daily Intake of Vitamins and Minerals

The Institute of Medicine (IOM) of the National Academy of Science (NAS) has determined, to the best of its ability, the amounts of vitamins and minerals that each individual needs every day from food plus supplements. No one who takes the "recommended amount" of any vitamin or mineral is known to suffer from a deficiency state (unless they have another medical problem causing it). Government agencies use different terms such as the Daily Value (DV) and Recommended Dietary Allowance (RDA). The Daily Value is the United States Food and Drug Administration's current term for how much of each vitamin and mineral to consume each day. Unfortunately, the Daily Values have not been updated for thirty years but are still used on the labels of vitamin bottles. The term Recommended Dietary Value was used previously. Don't let the changing nomenclature confuse you. Essentially, these terms mean the same thing.

Let's look at a table of twenty-seven vitamins and minerals. (You may remember that the Merck table listed twenty-eight nutrients but included fatty acids.) We can compare the Institute of Medicine's Recommended Amounts with the older U.S. Food and Drug Administration's Daily Values.[2] These values are for adults.

[2] Copyright 2006 CSPI. Reprinted from Nutrition Action Health Letter, March 2006. www.cspinet.org.

Vitamin	IOM Recommended Amount	Daily Value
Vitamin A (retinol)	3,000 IU	5,000 IU
Vitamin D	200 IU (adults under 50), 400 IU (adults 50–70), 600 – 1000 IU (adults over 70)	400 IU
Vitamin E	33 IU	30 IU
Vitamin K	120 mcg	80 mcg
Thiamin (B1)	1.2 mg	1.5 mg
Riboflavin (B2)	1.3 mg	1.7 mg
Niacin (B3)	16 mg	20 mg
Pyridoxine (B6)	1.7 mg	2.0 mg
Folic acid	400 mcg	400 mcg
Cobalamin (B12)	2.4 mcg	6 mcg
Vitamin C (ascorbic acid)	90 mg men, 75 mg women	60 mg
Biotin	30 mcg	300 mcg
Pantothenic acid	5 mg	10 mg
Potassium	4700 mg	3500 mg
Calcium	1000 mg if under 50, 1200 mg if over 50	1,000 mg
Phosphorous	700 mg	1,000 mg

Vitamin	IOM Recommended Amount	Daily Value
Magnesium	420 mg men, 320 women	400 mg
Iron	18 mg	18 mg
Iodine	150 mcg	150 mcg
Zinc	11 mg men, 8 mg women	15 mg
Copper	0.9 mg	2 mg
Chromium	35 mcg men, 25 mcg women	120 mcg
Selenium	55 mcg	70 mcg
Manganese	2.3 mg	2 mg
Molybdenum	45 mcg	75 mg
Chloride	2300 mg	3400 mg
Potassium	4700 mg	3500 mg

IU = International Units[3]

mg = milligrams. A milligram is 1/1000th of a gram.

mcg = micrograms. A microgram is 1/1000th of a milligram.

You can ignore these nutrients: biotin, pantothenic acid, iodine, manganese, molybdenum, chloride, and boron. Unless you eat a terrible diet, you need no more of these than you already obtain from your food.

The vast majority of people in advanced countries don't suffer deficiency states such as scurvy or rickets. If you obtain the above amounts, then you are assured of an adequate supply of the vitamins and minerals needed to maintain all the body's chemical processes.

While most of the values remain relatively constant between the two tables, some have changed. The IOM recommends 3,000 IU daily of Vitamin A while the older FDA Daily Value is 5,000 units. Can you get too much? Similarly, the IOM now recommends a daily intake of 90 mg of Vitamin C which is an increase from the FDA Daily Value of 60 mg. Which group should we believe? Are there some vitamins or minerals that, in high doses, can achieve beneficial effects in the body?

Some experts recommend huge doses of certain vitamins, com-

---

[3] International units (IU) are used to measure the effectiveness of a product, such as vitamins, minerals, hormones, and vaccines, within a biological system, such as the human body. The international unit was developed before science could accurately measure these products chemically. You can convert from IU to milligrams or micrograms. For example, 1 IU of Vitamin A = .6 mcg of beta-carotene or .3 mcg of retinol. These conversions tend to be confusing. Most vitamin manufacturers list Vitamins A, D, and E in IU and most other vitamins and minerals by weight (milligrams or micrograms).

monly called *mega doses*. Regarding the controversial Vitamin C, some nutritionists recommend from five hundred milligrams twice a day to a whopping twenty thousand milligrams a day. This philosophy got a tremendous boost when the Nobel Prize winner Dr. Linus Pauling recommended large doses of Vitamin C.

There are several problems with the recommendations for such high doses.

Dr. Pauling was not a nutritionist and virtually every researcher in the field since then has disagreed with him. As of this date, there is NO compelling evidence that massive doses of any vitamins cure anything. There are many vitamins and minerals that cause well-documented health problems if you consume too much of them. This is called *vitamin toxicity*. For example, hypervitaminosis A is well documented in medical literature. Excessive intake of Vitamin A can cause headache, enlarged spleen and liver, thickening of the bones, and peeling skin. You can check the Merck table in Chapter One to see those vitamins with a toxicity state. We know that high doses of some vitamins tend to interfere with the proper absorption of other vitamins. In addition, once inside the body, high doses of one vitamin can interfere with the healthy metabolic functioning of another.

Experts continue to argue over the ideal amount of different vitamins and minerals. Patients frequently get confused over these conflicting claims and, taking matters into their own hands, go to the pharmacy and pick out several bottles of their favorite vitamins and minerals without regard to the amounts contained in their diet. Here are my recommendations:

First, get an adequate amount of each vitamin and mineral daily. This can come from food or vitamin pills. Food is the preferred source since there are other compounds in food that are still being discovered that confer added health benefits. We'll talk about this more in Chapter Five.

Second, the IOM recommendations are more recent and probably more accurate and there fore should be used in preference to the older FDA values.

Third, there is no evidence taking extra amounts of any vitamin makes you healthier. Currently, the vitamin industry is a whopping $3 billion a year business in the United States. As one researcher wrote, this is an expensive way to color your urine. We'll devote an entire section in Chapter Five to discussing the pros and cons of taking vitamin pills if you already eat a healthy, balanced diet.

So, avoid <u>mega</u> doses of vitamins, especially those associated with a deficiency state. However, taking an <u>extra</u> dose of a vitamin with no toxicity state probably won't harm you. Let's cite an example.

The FDA Daily Value of Vitamin C is sixty milligrams. The IOM Daily Recommendation is ninety milligrams. You feel that Vitamin C cures the common cold. You note in the Merck table that there is no toxicity state associated with Vitamin C. Take two hundred to five hundred milligrams daily. Unless you're too sick to eat, obtain these extra doses from food: eat fruits and drink fruit juices that are rich in Vitamin C. Don't take thousands of milligrams of Vitamin C daily.

You'll learn which food groups contain the most of these vitamins and minerals in Chapter Five. Appendix C has extensive tables of nutrient values for many individual foods.

A Summary of the Chapter

One of the best ways to live a long, healthy life is to maintain a Desirable Body Weight. This is best determined from insurance tables, which are adjusted for your gender, height, and frame size. Regardless of your activity level, eating to maintain a healthy body weight will provide an adequate amount of calories for your energy needs.

Second, eat breakfast.

Third, eat regular meals.

Fourth, consume the IOM recommended amount of each vitamin and mineral daily. These nutrients allow the necessary chemical processes in our body to run smoothly and efficiently. We'll discuss individual food groups and their vitamin and mineral content in Chapter Five. Avoid mega doses of vitamins.

Fifth, follow the other advice in the Breslow Seven. Get regular exercise. Don't smoke. Use alcohol moderately, if at all. Get seven to eight hours of sleep a night.

Simple, huh?

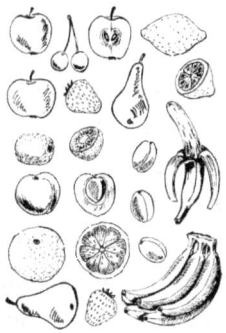

Chapter Three – Healthy Foods

Three Methods to Determine Healthy Foods

For this book, I have chosen three separate methods to determine which foods are the healthiest. We'll look at these methods, compare them, and decide what is consistent and advisable for us to apply to our own behavior. Please feel free to agree or disagree with my conclusions.

First, the United States government issues nutrition recommendations based on the latest research. Many people rely on this information as a guide to what to eat to maintain good health. The government updates these recommendations every five years.

The second method is to look at diets from different cultures whose people live a long time. These people are active and healthy well into their later years. Two cultures in particular have many members who live long and healthy lives, the Mediterranean and Japanese.

The third method is to look at the diet and lifestyle of two role models, in this case, two gentlemen. One is ninety-two years old and remains vigorous and active, with an energy level typical of individuals half his age. The other died recently at the age of one hundred after an incredible life. We'll see who they are shortly. Interestingly, in the United States, by the age of eighty-five, there are one hundred women for every forty men, making these two even more remarkable. However, our two role models have been chosen for their remarkable health and longevity, not for their gender.

"Why not rely only on research for your recommendations?" you may ask. Unfortunately, research is far from perfect. Most research in the field of nutrition deals with test tube experiments, animals, or a small group of individuals. These studies alone rarely provide convincing evidence for effectiveness in humans. Later researchers often disagree with the findings of previous studies, causing frequent confusion in the minds of the public. No wonder that patients say to me, "The scientists all disagree so I'll just eat what I want."

In the defense of science, we know that nutrition research is expensive, takes a long time, and is incredibly complex. Often, it's hard to tease out the benefits of any one food. The incredible variety of food available on the planet may contain a great number of ingredients, possibly over a hundred thousand different compounds, far more than previously realized.

In addition, people come from many cultures. Within any particular culture, individuals vary significantly. Besides genetics, a number of lifestyle factors are involved, such as smoking, alcohol, exercise, and even daily sunlight exposure. The real world outside the laboratory consists six billion of individuals with different genetic codes and family medical histories who are nurtured in thousands of different cultures.

In my opinion, research alone is insufficient. When we study individuals to see what they eat, how they act, how long they live, how healthy they are, and what diseases they die from, we can draw conclusions that are more valid and applicable to humans than the results of research done in a lab. We are most interested in lifestyle choices that healthy individuals and cultures make, to see if we can apply them to our own lives.

By examining and comparing each of these three methods, we can see if we find agreement as to what constitutes great nutrition. Then, we'll talk about four of the macronutrient groups that make up our diet: carbohydrate, protein, fat, and water. Also, to make it fun and, hopefully, easier to remember, I'll tell you about three groups called "The Good, The Bad, and The Ugly."

Method One – Key Recommendations From the Research

The Dietary Guidelines for Americans are published every five years as a joint effort by the United States Department of Health and Human Services (HHS) and the Department of Agriculture (USDA). They released the latest guidelines in 2005.

The following is a summary of their key recommendations:

1.) Choose a balanced diet.
2.) Include a variety of nutritious foods and beverages chosen from among the basic food groups.
3.) Limit the intake of saturated fats, trans fats, cholesterol, added sugars, salt, and alcohol.
4.) Stay within your energy needs. (The government uses a 2,000 calorie diet as a reference for most Americans).

The HHS and USDA encourage the following food intake:

1.) Consume two cups of fruit and two and one-half cups of vegetables each day. Choose a variety of each group. In particular, choose from among the five vegetable groups, which are dark green, orange, legumes, starchy vegetables, and other vegetables.
2.) At least half of your grains should come from whole grains, with a minimum of three ounces of whole grains daily.
3.) Consume three cups per day of fat-free milk, low fat milk, or equivalent dairy products.
4.) Consume less than 10 percent of calories from saturated fatty acids and less than 300 mg/day of cholesterol. Keep *trans* fatty acid consumption as low as possible.
5.) Keep total fat intake between 20 %to 35% of calories, with most fats coming from sources of polyunsaturated and monounsaturated fatty acids, such as fish, nuts, and vegetable oils.
6.) When selecting and preparing meat, poultry, dry beans, and milk or milk products, make choices that are lean, low-fat, or fat-free.
7.) Limit intake of fats and oils high in saturated or *trans* fatty acids. Choose products low in such fats and oils.
8.) Choose fiber-rich fruits, vegetables, and whole grains.
9.) Choose and prepare foods and beverages with little added sugars or caloric sweeteners.
10.) Reduce the incidence of dental cavities by practicing good oral hygiene and consuming less sugar- and starch-containing foods and beverages.

Method Two – Wonder Diets From Two Different Cultures

There has been a lot of press in the last few years regarding the "wonder" diets, those used by various cultures whose people enjoy long lives and who also have low rates of the two major killers, cancer and heart attacks. The two most popular diets are the *Mediterranean diet*, used on Crete and other Greek islands, and the *Japanese diet*, consumed in Okinawa and throughout much of Japan. Let's summarize each of these diets and also look briefly at the activity level of their members.

The Mediterranean Diet

The Mediterranean diet is primarily vegetarian. The people on the island of Crete eat lots of vegetables, including eggplant and mushrooms. These Greeks consume bean dishes with condiments and whole grain bread dipped in olive oil. They eat non-animal proteins such as lentils, nuts, peas, and beans daily, have a glass of a local wine with the meal, and often finish with fruit. On average, they eat fish two to three times a week, lamb and chicken each once a week.

The Mediterranean diet may contain as much as forty percent fat. The main source is olive oil, monounsaturated oil. Olive oil and whole grains accounted for half of their total calories. Meat, especially red meat, is much less common in the Mediterranean diet than in a typical American diet, as are dairy products, such as cheese and yogurt. Fish is much more common.

They are active physically. They walk to work. Many jobs entail hard or constant physical labor. Typical occupations include shepherd, farmer, olive grower, beekeeper, and fisherman. Many laborers burn 3,500 to 5,000 calories daily, far higher than the 1,500 to 2,000 calories that more sedentary individuals burn in an average day.

The Japanese Diet

The Japanese diet primarily consists of rice, vegetables, tofu, and fish. Land for grazing animals is scarce and expensive in Japan. The country's population is sixty percent the size of the U.S. population. The Japanese live in an area roughly the size of California. Due to the rarity and expense of cattle, they eat virtually no meat or dairy products.

Japan consists of four major islands surrounded by the ocean. Typical of the Japanese in general, people on Okinawa consume a tremendous amount of fish. Snacks such as cake, pastry, and cookies are rare. They drink a lot of green tea. The Japanese diet contains only ten percent total fat, with an incredibly low three percent coming from saturated fat. The Japanese eat rice at virtually every meal and consume tofu frequently. Obesity is extremely rare, unless you study a group of Sumo wrestlers. Regarding lifestyle, many Japanese people, like their Mediterranean counterparts, work agrarian jobs that require intense physical labor. Even those who work in the city often walk or bicycle extensively due to the congestion caused by the high concentration of people and cars in urban areas.

Historically, neither the Greeks nor the Japanese have taken vitamins. The Greek and Japanese populations consume a diet low in saturated fat and containing lots of fruits, vegetables, whole grains, and fish. They eat little red meat or dairy products. They seldom eat foods high in sugar. The Greeks consume red wine modestly with meals; the Japanese drink lots of green tea. Many members of both groups engage in regular strenuous physical activity, usually as part of their work, sometimes as a way to commute. We can assume that the Greeks get lots of sunlight, due to their occupations and the proximity of their country to the equator. The Japanese are farther north and therefore more distant from the equator. However, they probably get significant sunlight due to their agrarian economy, which requires outdoor work.

When we look at disease prevalence in these two cultures, we see that both the Greek and Japanese people have lower rates of heart disease than Westerners. They also have lower rates of several types of cancer, including prostate, breast, and colon cancer. Research studies in the West have implicated a high fat diet in all three types of cancer.

Method Three – Exceptional Individuals

My first gentleman is ninety-five years old. He lives in California. In 1984, on his seventieth birthday, he swam in Long Beach Harbor with his wrists handcuffed and his feet shackled, towing seventy rowboats with one person in each for one and a half miles. Few people could perform this feat at any age, let alone at the age of seventy.

Until the age of fifteen, he was addicted to sugar, "a junk food junkie," in his own words. Then he went to hear a pioneer nutritionist named Paul Bragg speak at the Oakland City Women's Club. Paul promised that anyone who exercised and ate a proper diet could achieve good health. So the young gentleman found a local YMCA with a set of weights and began exercising.

Doctors warned him against weight lifting. "You can weaken the heart," they said. "You'll have a heart attack." They even threatened, "You'll lose your sex drive." At that time, coaches felt that their athletes would become muscle bound if they worked out with weights. In spite of these dire warnings, he continued.

He states, "My top priority in life is my workout each day." He typically gets up between four and five in the morning to exercise for two hours. He also swims everyday.

He read Gray's Anatomy voraciously, beginning a lifelong practice of reading books and articles on nutrition and exercise. He also earned a chiropractic degree to learn more about the body.

Who is our mystery man? None other than Jack La Lanne, long considered America's Number One Fitness Guru and the Godfather of Physical Fitness.[1] Jack has been in business for seventy years, since 1936, when he opened the country's first modern health center. His television show aired in 1951 and his popular fitness program ran for a record thirty-four years. Jack finds it gratifying to see that everything he was preaching over fifty years ago regarding both exercise and nutrition has come to fruition. "Back then I was a crackpot, today I am an authority. And believe me, I can't die. It would ruin my image."

One of his favorite sayings is, "If the mind can conceive, the body can achieve."

What about nutrition? After hearing the nutritionist Paul Bragg speak, Jack ate a vegetarian diet for a short time. However, for the next sixty years or so, he ate a much broader variety of foods, including the following:

- Whole grains, including brown rice, potatoes, and 100% whole wheat
- Fruits

---

[1] Thanks to the La Lannes for their kind permission to include this description and for adding a few comments of their own.

- Vegetables
- Low-fat dairy food
- Fish
- Lean meat, including chicken and turkey

Jack also frequently supplemented his diet with wheat germ and brewer's yeast. In fact, he wrote that he liked to supplement every meal this way. He ate honey instead of sugar. He states emphatically that fat is the killer.

Jack ate little white bread or beef. He wisely gave up foods that are no longer recommended, such as liver, an organ meat that is high in saturated fat and often containing toxins filtered from the animal's blood stream.

What does he eat now?

For breakfast, Jack has a shake containing vitamins, minerals, and proteins. He also has a soy drink with fifty grams of protein.

For lunch, Jack has four egg whites from hard boiled eggs or an egg white omelet plus five pieces of fruit. He may add a juicer drink containing lots of fruits and vegetables from the refrigerator.

For dinner, Jack has a salad with ten different raw vegetables, fish, brown rice, and a soup with no cream.

So, Jack's diet has evolved. He is unafraid to consult a nutritionist.

During an interview with Dateline NBC in the fall of 2002, Jack stated that he gave up drinking milk, feeling that it is meant for suckling calves, not humans. (As we will see, cow's milk remains controversial among nutritionists to this day, with some stating that it's essential to a healthy diet and an excellent source of calcium, while others claim that cow's milk is poorly digested and shouldn't be consumed by humans).

Jack also told the interviewers that he hadn't eaten junk food in seventy years. Yes, that's right, seventy years. He eats no hot dogs, cookies, cake, or soda pop. None.

Previously, at the age of eighty-five, Jack told the same Dateline interviewers that he didn't need Viagra. They had trouble believing him. However, his claim makes sense. If you maintain your overall fitness through nutrition and exercise, your entire body stays young. The blood vessels remain open and vigorous, delivering well-oxygenated and nutrient-rich blood to all parts of the body.

If you want to keep an eye on his progress, Jack's birthday is September 26, 1914. He'll be one hundred years old in the year 2014. Let's hope that he's still appearing on television to explain his vision of health.

We turn now to a second gentleman who died in 2003 at the age of one hundred. He was a senator in the United States Congress for an incredible forty-eight years. This man was re-elected in 1997 to the Senate from South Carolina. He finished his last term of office in 2003 after becoming the oldest person ever to sit in Congress at the age of one hundred.

At the age of sixty-six, this man married a twenty-one year old beauty queen against the advice of many of his political advisors who felt that the marriage might ruin his political career. The couple had four children together, two boys and two girls, long before there was medication for impotence.

Who accomplished all this? In case you haven't already guessed, it was Senator Strom Thurmond.

What were Senator Thurmond's secrets about such a long and productive life? I talked to his secretary on the telephone about his lifestyle on April 28, 1993. She told me that the Senator exercised one hour a day, seven days a week. Until he was eighty-six, Thurmond jogged every morning, after which his doctor told him to switch to a stationary bicycle because it was safer. His exercise regimen included calisthenics, stretching, sit-ups, and pull-ups. He performed the sit-ups with his arms crossed over his chest, knees bent, and feet under the couch. He did standard pushups. After quitting jogging, Thurmond spent twenty minutes on the stationary bicycle. He then lifted weights. He swam three to four times a week for one hour in the evening. The Senator was fond of saying, "You got to circulate the blood." Since the man also ran cross-country in college at Clemson, he exercised for over eighty years, longer than most people live.

What about nutrition? The Senator avoided fried foods and sugar. He ate a lot of fruits, vegetables, fish, and lean chicken. He had Jell-O every night "for his fingernails," feeling that the gelatin kept the nails strong. He took a vitamin supplement and a fiber supplement.

The Senator wasn't a teetotaler but drank an occasional beer. He was strongly opposed to smoking.

He did well without a lot of sleep. He worked past midnight and often sent his office workers home early to get their rest. He tolerated stress well.

His philosophy was "don't dwell on the past," and "work on things you can change." Thurmond met the positive-thinking gurus Napoleon Hill and Clement Stone. He read a lot, especially news magazines and politics, just to keep up with his field.

A few days after my call to the secretary, a letter arrived from the Senator.[2] The text is as follows:

April 28, 1993
Dear Dr. Grusenmeyer:

Thank you for your inquiry regarding my daily health and fitness routine. It was good of you to take the time to write.

Since exercise and good nutrition are the keys to good health, I follow a strict fitness program and diet. I avoid foods high in fat and sugar, and eat lots of fruits and vegetables, as well as whole-grain products and low-fat protein like fish.

I exercise every morning for approximately an hour. My workout includes 20 minutes of calisthenics, 20 minutes on a stationary bicycle and 10 or 20 minutes of weightlifting. I also swim ½ mile several times a week. I have exercised all my life. As a child, I worked on my parents' farm, walked a long way to school and enjoyed horseback riding. Later, I ran track and played other sports in high school and college.

In addition to sound nutrition and exercise, a good mental attitude is important to a healthy lifestyle. I believe that helping others and keeping an optimistic attitude about life are essential to achieving good mental health.

Thank you again for your interest, and with kindest regards and best wishes,

Sincerely,
Strom Thurmond

---

[2]Reprinted with the kind permission of the Thurmond family and estate.

As we noted, this gentleman served for forty-eight years in the United States Senate and lived to the age of one hundred, both marvelous feats. Yet, in my opinion, he may have lived longer had his life not been marred by tragedy. In May, 1993, less than one month after he wrote the letter you just read, his twenty-two year-old daughter, Nancy Moore Thurmond, was run down and killed by a drunken driver. According to news reports, her father, ninety years old at the time, grieved her loss tremendously. Perhaps, just as calm and tranquility add to our health and longevity, tragedy and sorrow subtract from them.

So, in a nutshell, what did he eat?

- Fruits
- Vegetables
- Whole grains
- Fish

He avoided fried foods and foods high in fat and sugar.

He never smoked. He exercised for an hour every morning and swam several times a week. He avoided stress and took a positive mental attitude.

Comparison of the Three Methods

Can we find agreement among our three sources of information? Or is all the evidence contradictory, confusing, or unhelpful?

To my way of thinking, a clear and consistent picture begins to emerge. The Greek and Japanese diets do agree with most epidemiological studies performed in the United States. If we look at the government summary of the research, the Mediterranean and Japanese diets, and the diet of our two role models, we can draw several conclusions.

First, a plant-based diet, which includes lots of fruits, vegetables, and whole grains, is conducive to good health. Second, saturated fat, sugar, and red meat should be eaten in moderation or not at all. Third, fish is a beneficial component of a balanced diet.

As an aside, the American Heart Association recently recommended that patients consume one gram of omega-3 fatty acids per day, preferably from fish rather than supplements. This amount is contained in a three ounce serving of fish such as salmon, herring, trout, or sardines, or a six ounce serving of canned tuna, halibut, or flounder. If you have high triglycerides, the American Heart Association recommends two to four grams per day from supplements. Supplements may also help patients with psoriasis, rheumatoid arthritis, and other autoimmune disorders.

Some epidemiologists, scientists who study the prevalence of disease, have drawn further conclusions which appear less consistent. Red wine, green tea, and tofu may provide some benefit. Note that not all of the above groups used these foods. The Japanese drink lots of green tea and eat lots of tofu. The Greeks drink a small glass of red wine several times a week.

We'll address the red wine and green tea issue more thoroughly in Chapter Six.

Are There Any Other Common Threads?

Are there other components, not related to nutrition, that all three methods have in common? Are there other lessons that we can learn from our three sources? While we continue to emphasize that our health is based on many factors, I feel comfortable making the following further recommendations.

First, stay physically active. A growing body of medical research indicates that exercise is a vital ingredient in maintaining health and vitality. Interestingly, both of our role models exercised vigorously for one to two hours daily for over seventy years. Jack La Lanne continues to exercise to this day. The people of both cultures we looked at work agrarian jobs and maintain a high level of physical activity throughout their lives.

Second, avoid stress. A stressful lifestyle is a killer. High stress has been linked to heart attack, stroke, a weakened immune system, and early death. High stress isn't prevalent in Greece and Japan. In these countries, as in many agrarian societies, the family unit is close. Crime is low. The local community is strong and supportive. This stable lifestyle contributes to the development of a peaceful climate for human growth. Both of our role models actively practice altruism. Senator Thurmond worked for years as a public servant. Mr. La Lanne taught fitness for decades. Each read books on positive thinking. Jack La Lanne's books are filled with advice about getting along with other people. He recommends performing acts of kindness and frequently encourages people to donate blood. Should you wish to read more about this remarkable man, consult his books *The Jack La Lanne Way to Vibrant Health* or *For Men Only*, which has excellent advice for both genders. His enthusiasm for the healthy lifestyle leaps from every page. You will find it contagious.

Third, don't smoke. The evidence against smoking is overwhelming.

Fourth, drink moderately or not at all. A glass of wine a day may confer some health benefits but research is devastating in its conclusions about heavy drinking. Heavy alcohol consumption interferes with body metabolism, destroys brain cells, weakens bones, slows reflexes, contributes to increased violent and hazardous behavior, breaks up families, consumes needed financial resources, clouds judgment, and interferes with thinking in general. Alcohol in excess devastates lives.

Our role models and our cultures either do not drink at all (such as Jack La Lanne, the Japanese diet) or drink very moderately (Strom Thurmond, the Greek diet).

So, there it is: Eat healthy. Exercise. Learn to reduce or deal with stress. Don't smoke. Drink moderately or not at all.

Gosh, this sounds a lot like the Breslow Seven.

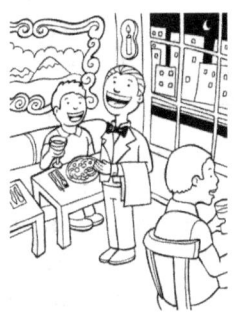

Chapter Four -
Food: The Good, the Bad, and the Ugly

Introduction

This chapter is designed for readers in a hurry. In it, you'll find short lists of foods that are healthy and unhealthy. You'll also find brief instructions on how to read a label. Last, we'll talk about fast food restaurants. I'll have suggestions for the daunting task of finding good nutrition there.

Chapter Five goes into greater detail on individual food groups.

Recall that we obtain all of our energy from three sources: carbohydrates, proteins, and fats. We can apply what we've learned in Chapter Three to find good and bad choices in each group. Remember that most foods have a combination of the three macro nutrients in them. One will often predominate, so the food will be listed under its predominant constituent. In each, I'll make specific suggestions for what to eat and what to avoid.

Good and Bad Carbohydrate

Recall that HDL is the "healthy cholesterol." High levels of HDL have been linked to clean arteries and a lower rate of heart attack and stroke. On the other hand, high total cholesterol and specifically LDL, the "lousy cholesterol," have been linked to hardening of the arteries and a higher rate of cardiovascular disease such as heart attack and stroke. Optimally a healthy diet maximizes the level of HDL in the bloodstream and minimizes the level of total and LDL cholesterol. Whole grains, particularly oats, have been shown to improve HDL.

Total cholesterol and LDL are higher if you consume a diet consisting mostly of processed grains.

Let's explain the difference.

Refined flour is made by removing the kernel's bran and germ. *Bran* is the husk or skin of grains such as wheat, rye, and oats. Bran is rich in fiber but is the byproduct of the milling of these grains. *Germ* refers to the nutrient-rich kernel of grains. Processed grains have been stripped of most vitamins and fiber. Can you think of a better way to ruin a food? The manufacturers then add four synthetic vitamins and minerals and call this flour "enriched."

Unfortunately, refined flour is ubiquitous in advanced civilizations. Refined flour is used to make virtually all pasta, noodles, cakes, cookies, crackers, bread, bagels, pizza dough, pretzels, cereals, donuts, and other snack foods. In the United States, we live in a "bleached white flour" country where most of the healthy fiber, vitamins, and minerals have been removed before the food is made.

Looking for food made with "unbleached flour" won't help. Unbleached simply means that the manufacturer hasn't bleached, or colored, the flour – but it is still stripped of its healthy components.

What should you look for when you buy any food containing grains? In two words - whole grains. The government's recommendation that "at least half of your grains should be whole grains" is an improvement over previous advice but doesn't go far enough. If possible, *all* of the grains you eat should be whole grains. By law, the ingredients on a food label must be listed in decreasing order by weight. Look for labels that list a whole grain as the first ingredient. Look for the words "whole wheat," or "whole oats," or "whole grain corn," or "bran" as the first ingredient. Ideally, the whole grain should be the only type of flour in the bread or cereal.

You can also look for the amount of fiber in the food. Bread made from whole grains is high in fiber. A slice of bread made with refined white flour will have one gram or less of fiber; a slice of bread made with whole grain flour will have three or more grams of fiber.

People who eat at least seven grams of bran a day have a thirty percent lower risk of coronary artery disease than those who consume no bran. Bran cereals pack an impressive twenty grams of fiber per cup, as opposed to seven to ten grams per cup of other healthy cereal and a pitiful zero to three grams of fiber in the "junk cereals," those made mostly from bleached flour and sugar. Generally, bran cereals contain much more bran than bran bread. Bran muffins vary tremendously in their bran content so you may want to read the label or ask the baker.

Don't let the names of different types of fiber confuse you. For example, oats, peas, and beans all contain the soluble fiber beta-glucans. Apples contain the soluble fiber pectin. Wheat bran contains the insoluble fibers lignin and cellulose. You can disregard these unfamiliar names. You may even disregard the differences between soluble and insoluble fiber. If you eat a variety of whole grains, fruits, and vegetables, you'll get plenty of both kinds of fiber. We'll talk about this more in the next chapter.

What are the healthy carbohydrates? Here is a list:

1.) Whole grains
2.) Fruits
3.) Vegetables
4.) Beans. There are no bad beans.

What are the bad carbohydrates?

1.) Starches, including all breads, cereals, crackers, and pasta (macaroni, spaghetti, and so on), donuts, and bagels made with processed flour. Avoid all of these "white bread" products.

2.) Sweets – cake, cookies, candy.

These foods contain mostly sugar (often the first ingredient), highly processed white flour, and hydrogenated vegetable oil – all three bad choices.

3.) French fries and potatoes, especially if you load them with items high in saturated fat, such as sour cream, butter, cheese, and most sauces.

Good and Bad Protein

Healthy protein includes lean meats and fish which are low in saturated fat. Try the following protein-rich foods:

1.) Turkey breast
2.) Chicken breast

3.) Fish, especially those high in omega-3 fatty acids, including salmon, sardines, and tuna. Some fish, especially the larger predators in the food chain, are high in mercury. These include swordfish, shark, tile fish, and king mackerel.

4.) Soybeans. Like all foods, the closer to nature, the better they are for you, or, to state the corollary, the less processed, the better. Nature, not the manufacturer, makes what is healthiest. First try unsalted whole soybeans or roasted soy nuts, then tofu. Soy milks and other more processed forms of soy contain lots of added ingredients and less soy.

You may ask, "Aren't soybeans a carbohydrate?" Actually, soybeans contain all three macro nutrients. They have about 13 grams of protein, 11 grams of carbohydrate, and 7 grams of fat per 100 gram portion. Since protein is the major constituent, soy beans are listed here.

Unhealthy proteins are high in saturated fat. Meat is a protein but often contains large amounts of fat. Avoid the following:

1.) Fatty meats usually made from processed pork – bacon, sausage, pepperoni, hot dogs, and cold cuts such as bologna and salami.

2.) Fatty beef. Prime rib, for example, often served an inch thick and twelve inches wide, contains huge deposits of fat marbled through the meat.

You'll read more about this in the section entitled "The Ugly," which contains lots of fatty processed meats.

Good and Bad Fat

As noted, we need fats in the diet. Although we need some fat to thrive, there are healthy diets that contain minimal fat and almost no saturated fat, such as the Japanese diet and Jack La Lanne's diet. To return to an earlier image, saturated fat clogs the arteries, like pouring lard down your kitchen sink clogs the pipes in the household plumbing. Physiologically, few goals are more important than getting a healthy, nutrient-rich blood supply to all our cells. If you keep your arteries open and clean, you improve your chances lf living a longer, healthier life.

My advice is that you take great care in the choice of fats that you add to your diet.

Healthy fats include the following:

1.) Nuts

    Almonds
    Brazil nuts*
    Cashews*
    Hazelnuts
    Macadamias*
    Peanuts
    Pecans
    Pine nuts, pignola
    Pine nuts, pinyon*
    Pistachios
    Walnuts

    * = higher in saturated fat.

Most of the nuts contain one to two grams of saturated fat per ounce. However, Brazil nuts, cashews, macadamias, and pinyon pine nuts contain three to five grams of saturated fat per ounce. They are noted with an asterisk in the table. Eat less of them, especially if you are watching your weight. Hazelnuts, pecan, pine nuts, and peanuts are a better choice since they are high in monounsaturated fat.

Nuts are a powerhouse of nutrients. Most are rich in calcium, iron, magnesium, phosphorous, potassium, zinc, and manganese, along with some selenium, copper and niacin. Almonds are high in Vitamin E and omega-3 fatty acids, cashews are high in Vitamin K, and pistachios are high in Vitamin A. None contain Vitamin B_{12} or Vitamin D.

My recommendation is that you eat a variety of unsalted nuts with no added oil. You'll find a complete table of nutrients for nuts in Appendix C.

2.) Olives
3.) Avocados
4.) Fish high in Omega-3 fatty acids

Growing evidence shows that foods rich in omega-3 fatty acids protect the heart and blood vessels. These fatty acids are linked to lower triglycerides, decreased clotting tendency, and lower risks of arrhythmia and sudden death. They are found in the following:

1.) Salmon, tuna, shrimp, squid, halibut, herring, rainbow trout, anchovies
2.) Flaxseed
3.) Walnuts
4.) Canola and soybean oils.

The following items are high in saturated fat or trans fat - avoid them:

1.) Lard and all kinds of animal fats
2.) Butter, cream, cheese, whole milk
3.) Hydrogenated vegetable oil, vegetable shortening
4.) Palm, palm kernel, and coconut oil; coconut meat

Summary: The Good, the Bad, and the Ugly

Some patients remember foods better if they have a slogan. Here are my choices for those foods that fit the categories of Good, Bad, and Ugly:

The Good

Good foods are high in vitamins, minerals, fiber, and antioxidants, low in cholesterol and saturated fat and contain no trans fat. Eat these in abundance:

1.) Fruit. All fruits and fruit juices are good, but emphasize the fruit rather than the juice. If you drink juice, try to find "juice not from concentrate." The more pulp that the juice contains, the higher its fiber content will be.
2.) All vegetables. Some states now have a slogan about fruits and vegetables, "Eat Five to Stay Alive." Some researchers now recommend ten a day. Varying the colors is an excellent suggestion, eating some vegetables that are yellow, orange, green, and purple. The new slogan is, "Five a day the color way." A robust salad will contain many of the colors of the rainbow. No fruits or vegetables contain cholesterol. The only fruits or vegetables that contain fat are coconuts,

olives, and avocados. Coconut meat is high in saturated fat, a rare occurrence in plant-based foods. Olives and avocados have monounsaturated fat, the healthy kind, so these foods are a good source for the fat necessary in a balanced diet. Generally, the more colorful the fruits or vegetables, the more vitamins and minerals they contain. Look for the colorful produce.

3.) All whole grains. Find these in breads and cereals.

4.) Legumes. What are legumes? A legume is a plant bearing a pod. That means peas and beans.

5.) Nuts.

6.) Fish (especially sardines, salmon, shellfish).

As seen in the results of the Mediterranean and Japanese diets, eating fish as a regular part of your diet is advantageous in numerous ways.

7.) Low-fat dairy products, like yogurt, skim milk, and 1% milk. Dairy products remain one of the few controversial areas in nutrition. We'll discuss them at length in the next chapter on specific foods.

8.) Soy, especially whole soy products.

And remember, the less processed the food, the better. Mother Nature knows our bodies far better than any food manufacturer.

The Bad

The first four foods are high in saturated fat. The fifth fills children's bellies, providing lots of calories from sugar while providing no vitamins, minerals, or fiber. Can you guess what it is? Here are my choices for bad foods:

1.) Coconut oil.

2.) Palm oil.

Coconut oil and palm oil are high in saturated fat but unfortunately are among the cheapest oils, making them a favorite of manufacturers. They are found in snacks including pastries, cookies, and movie popcorn.

3.) Likewise, *hydrogenated* vegetable oil is high in saturated fat. Check the ingredient label to find this hidden item.

4.) High-fat dairy products, like cream, butter, and cheese. All are high in saturated fat.

As an aside, many of my patients are quite proud of their diet, especially claiming that they eat little fat. I often walk through the list of high-fat foods with them and they proudly deny eating them. Some of them have trouble losing weight. I will often say, "Now I can predict your downfall. I'll bet you eat a lot of cheese." Ninety percent of the time patients react by saying, "You're kidding! I had no idea that cheese was high in fat."

The three highest sources of fat intake for Americans are: first, cheese; second, whole milk; and third, beef. So, if you love dairy products, consider eating small amounts of low-fat cheese, skim or 1% milk.

Butter is loaded with saturated fat. Why not skip the spread? Eat your bread plain or, if you wish, with a little fruit or honey. If you choose jam or jelly, choose a variety whose first ingredient is fruit, preferably a sugar-free brand. But you really don't need any spread. If you eat your bread plain, you can rediscover the savory, crunchy, delicious taste of whole grains.

5.) Soda pop. You may have guessed this last entry. Soda is not technically a food but a manufacturer's concoction consisting of water, corn syrup, artificial colors, flavors, and usually caffeine. Thus, the terms *empty calories* and *nutritional bankruptcy* describe this non-food. You get the calories you need as fuel but without any of the vitamins, minerals, or fiber found in healthy food. Also, 100% of the calories come from sugar or, more commonly, the inexpensive substitute, corn sweetener, a carbohydrate. Malnourished children in poorer areas of the United States often get enough calories but derive a great proportion of them from nutritionally bankrupt foods like soda pop.

Incredibly, the soda manufacturers in the United States make enough soft drinks to provide every man, woman, and child with over 500 twelve-ounce cans per year. Approximately sixty percent of all Americans drink soda every day. Thus, one of our greatest sources of calories is a nutritionally bankrupt liquid.

The Ugly

What food is considered harmful to the human species? Why have I singled out these foods as particularly bad?

Most of the top ten worst foods are high in lard. *Lard* is pure animal fat. Some of the worst foods also contain lots of trans fat, another artery clogger. Many of these ugly foods, including number one through five, are commonly cured with nitrites, a preservative which has been associated with cancer of the colon. These foods are extremely high in salt, which is a no-no for anyone with high blood pressure. Most are also high in calories. Remember that fat contains nine calories per gram compared to four calories per gram for carbohydrate and protein, making these food especially harmful choices for anyone trying to lose weight.

Here are some really ugly foods:

1.) Bacon. When you buy a pound of bacon, all of the white part is lard. The factory places the part containing the most red meat toward the little plastic window in the front of the package. Don't be fooled.

2.) Pepperoni. Last year, a local pizza parlor advertised their special of the week - a large pizza with double cheese and triple pepperoni. They actually sent a flyer to houses in the neighborhood bragging about this item. Their promotional slogan was "Try a heart attack in a box." At least they were honest. They can't be accused of false advertising. You might as well just lather your arteries with grease.

3.) Sausage.

4.) Lunchmeat (bologna, salami, other cold cuts of meat).

5.) Hot dogs.

6.) Organ meats (liver, kidney, brain, tongue). Although liver is a good source of iron and Vitamin A, it is high in cholesterol and saturated fat. Also, the liver filters many of the toxins from the animal's body. So, the drawbacks of liver outweigh its benefits. There are many better sources of Vitamin A.

7.) Most pork, or meat from the pig, including ham. (Pork is not "the other white meat." Beef, pork, and lamb are all <u>red</u> meat.) Many cuts of pork are loaded with fat. (See items Number 1 through 5). Pork is simply not as lean as chicken or turkey, the two white meats.

8.) Potato chips, which are mostly fat and salt covering a wafer-thin slice of potato. You eat very little potato, which is not a good starch choice anyway. Sweet potatoes and yams are far more nutritious.

9.) Doughnuts are another killer. They are superb at increasing your waist size and adding plaque to the arteries. Doughnuts consist of bleached white flour, hydrogenated oil, and sugar mixed together and deep fried in more oil loaded with trans fat. To assure the complete destruction of your youthful fig-ure, the manufacturers often fill the center of the doughnut with cream or jelly. The cream is virtually all sugar. Can you guess how much fruit is in the jelly?

Here are some statistics to wrap your mouth around. A single doughnut contains 200 to 350 calories, one to six grams of trans fat, plus two to ten grams of saturated fat. Yes, that's in <u>each</u> doughnut. If you eat half a dozen dough-nuts, you're talking 1,200 to 2,100 calories, six to thirty-six grams of trans fat, and twelve to sixty grams of saturated fat. That's why you need to sit down and rest after eating this amount - your blood is sluggish.

Perhaps we can call a dozen doughnuts "a coma in a box."

10.) French fries, especially those cooked in lard. French fries can contain a whopping two hundred calories derived from fat in a single serving. Whew.

I worked at McDonald's during high school. Back then, we cooked the fries in lard. The lard came in a big block that measured two feet square. We struggled to get the big cube out of its tin container and into the vat of frying oil. Today, most companies use a low-fat vegetable oil to cook fries, which helps to reduce the fat and calorie content.

Unfortunately, the product is still high in both calories and fat. Often the fries come loaded with salt, compliments of the fast food worker with the giant salt shaker, who liberally pours salt on your favorite food before you can say, "hold the high blood pressure."

11.) Junk cereals, which are high in sugar, processed flour, plus artificial food coloring, flavors, and preservatives. You don't want to serve this to your children. Junk cereals contain processed grains (usually wheat, especially our old nemesis, "bleached white flour"). Children are the primary consumers of these products, victims of a savvy Saturday morning advertising campaign on television.

12.) The bacon double cheeseburger. This sandwich actually contains four high-fat ingredients: bacon, beef, cheese, and mayonnaise. The average burger contains a whopping amount of fat - forty to seventy grams. Mayonnaise is responsible for seventeen of those fat grams.

If the double cheese, triple pepperoni pizza is a heart attack in a box, the bacon double cheeseburger qualifies for "a stroke in a box." If you eat two, you can have one for each of the carotid arteries, those large vessels in the neck that supply blood to the brain.

13.) Meat-lovers pizza. This is a high-fat food, made with our old friend refined flour covered with loads of high-fat cheese and the unhealthiest meats, such as sausage, bacon, and pepperoni. The only redeeming items are the calcium in the cheese, which you can get elsewhere, and a thin layer of tomato sauce. Some of these pizzas contain five items high in saturated fat – sausage, bacon, ground beef, pepperoni, and cheese. You won't find vegetables in a meat-lovers pizza.

14.) Twisted salted beef. This concoction is mostly saturated fat, fried grease, and salt, with a generous helping of sodium nitrite, a preservative. If you really want to eat this food, just check the ingredients on the label before putting it in your mouth. Is it any wonder that this food often contains the word "jerky?"

Don't panic. There is good news for junk food fans. You don't have to give up all the foods that you love. Just think of healthier varieties of the same foods. For example, if you like pizza, try this: Use whole-grain flour, a small amount of low-fat cheese, and lots of tomato sauce. Make it a vegetarian pizza, loaded with vegetable toppings. Add green olives, onions, mushrooms, and artichokes. If you're adventurous, you can even add broccoli. Skip the meat entirely.

Now, that's a real pizza. Your arteries will dance for joy, you won't feel lethargic afterward, and you'll get lots of vitamins, minerals, anti-oxidants, and fiber, with almost no fat. Your waist line will shrink accordingly. Even if you don't love vegetables now, you can develop a taste for them. You'll feel better after eating this type of pizza rather than a "heart attack in a box."

Instead of a doughnut, why not grab a bran muffin? If you buy muffins, make sure that they're high in fiber and contain no trans fat and minimal saturated fat. Better yet, why not make your own? If you're too busy, how about cutting out one hour of television per week?

How to Read Labels

Reading food labels is crucial and can be simple. Healthy eaters rarely choose any food without scanning the label for a few seconds. Here is a sample food label from the Food and Drug Administration website:

The Nutrition Facts label contains vital information and is a good way of figuring out what you're eating. However, these labels confuse many people. Let's go over a commonsense, easy guide to reading a nutrition label. Essentially, you only need to look at seven simple items to tell how healthy the food is and what happened at the factory.

Nutrition Facts

Serving Size 1 cup (228g)
Servings Per Container 2

Amount Per Serving

Calories 250	Calories from Fat 110

	% Daily Value*
Total Fat 12g	18%
Saturated Fat 3g	15%
Trans Fat 1.5g	
Cholesterol 30mg	10%
Sodium 470mg	20%
Total Carbohydrate 31g	10%
Dietary Fiber 0g	0%
Sugars 5g	
Protein 5g	

Vitamin A	4%
Vitamin C	2%
Calcium	20%
Iron	4%

* Percent Daily Values are based on a 2,000 calorie diet. Your Daily Values may be higher or lower depending on your calorie needs:

	Calories:	2,000	2,500
Total Fat	Less than	65g	80g
Sat Fat	Less than	20g	25g
Cholesterol	Less than	300mg	300mg
Sodium	Less than	2,400mg	2,400mg
Total Carbohydrate		300g	375g
Dietary Fiber		25g	30g

Seven Simple Suggestions

Let's work from top to bottom.

1.) Look at serving size, the first item on the label. Look at the familiar units, such as the number of cups or pieces. Ignore the amount in parentheses, listed in grams, unless you're familiar with the metric system.

Ask yourself, "How many servings am I eating?" If the serving size is one cup and you eat two cups, then double all the values in the table. Let's assume for this example that you are eating one serving.

2.) Look at calories, the next item on the label. Calories are energy or fuel, just like gasoline is fuel for your car. Excess calories turn into weight gain if we eat more than we burn off per day. So, if you're interested in keeping your weight down, a food with lots of calories per serving is not your best bet. On the same line is the entry calories from fat. Generally, the more calories there are from fat, the less healthy the food, although there are exceptions, such as nuts. So, let's look at the next item on the label.

3.) Total fat. Foods that are high in fat content really pack in the calories. So, the less total fat, the fewer calories. Some patients are confused on seeing that there are often several categories in this section. These include total fat, saturated fat, trans fat, monounsaturated fat, and polyunsaturated fat.

Just remember that saturated fat and trans fat clog the arteries. Here's an easy rule: minimal saturated fat and NO trans fat on every label. Monounsaturated and polyunsaturated fat are healthier choices. Foods that are high in these fats can be good for you.

4.) The next item is cholesterol. Look for foods that are low in cholesterol. The government recommends three hundred milligrams of cholesterol pr day in a balanced 2,000 calorie diet.

5.) The next item is sodium, one of the two ingredients in table salt. If you have high blood pressure, make sure that the sodium content is low.

Unfortunately, virtually all the packaged foods in the grocery store are loaded with sodium. As an intelligent buyer, what can you do?

Here are some options.

First, stick to the perimeter of the grocery store. You'll find produce, such as fresh fruits and vegetables, which contain zero to minimal amounts of salt. Second, if you buy packaged food, look for items that contain no salt, like frozen vegetables and many breakfast cereals. Many canned soups and vegetables are now labeled "Low Salt" or "Low Sodium." Third, avoid cured meats that are loaded with salt.

6.) The next item is fiber. Generally, the higher the fiber content, the healthier the food. Beans, fruits, vegetables, and whole grain all contain lots of fiber. Ideally, look for three grams of fiber or more per serving.

7.) The last item is sugar. Generally, unless you are starving or calorie deficient, the less sugar the better. The sugar you get from eating fruit will be more than sufficient.

On the right side of the Nutrition Facts label you'll read "% DV," which stands for "percent of daily value." Most nutritionists instruct their patients to ignore these values as they can be confusing. They're most helpful if you are calculating the percentage of a particular vitamin or mineral that you're getting in your diet each day.

At the bottom of the label is a footnote explaining percent daily value. You'll notice this just after the asterisk. Let's say that you want to make sure that you get 100% of your daily value of calcium each day. In the label above, the item contains 20% of the daily value of calcium. If you know that the daily value of calcium is 1200 mg, and you get 20% of that, then you are getting 20% times 1200 mg, or 240 mg. If you eat one serving, then you still need 80% of your daily value from other foods. If you eat two servings, making 40%, you still need 60% of your daily value of calcium from other foods. So, you still need to get 60% of 1200 mg, or 720 mg, to reach 100% of the daily value of calcium for the day.

This part of the label is the most confusing. Feel free to ignore it. If you wish to learn how to ensure that you get a proper amount of each vitamin and mineral in your daily diet, check Chapter Ten entitled, "How to be your Own Nutritionist."

Remember my promise in the Introduction to make difficult concepts easy? Perhaps you feel that the "Seven Simple Suggestions" aren't so simple. You'd like something easier and faster.

Just scan the list of ingredients. Make sure the first two to three ingredients are natural and healthy. Two quick rules apply. First, good foods contain only a few ingredients and you'll know them by name. Second, ingredients with long confusing names that you have trouble pronouncing are generally unhealthy – unless they are vitamins and minerals. By now you can pick these names out since you've scanned the Merck Table of Vitamins and Minerals. Put the items with lots of long, unrecognizable ingredients back on the shelf in favor of one with a short list of natural ingredients. One of my favorite cereals has one ingredient. The label says, "Whole grain wheat." Sweet.

Fast Food Restaurants

They don't call these joints "greasy spoons" for nothing. The menu offerings at fast food restaurants are quite high in calories, total fat, saturated fat, cholesterol, sugar, and sodium. Nutrients and fiber are sparse. The most nutritious foods, such as fruits, vegetables, whole grains, beans, and nuts are missing from the menu (in all fairness, you do get one or two pickle slices on a Big Mac). Before you buy, ask for a copy of their nutrition facts. See if you can find the healthy foods hiding on the list.

A single big hamburger at a particularly famous fast-food chain contains the following: 560 calories, thirty grams of total fat, including ten grams of saturated fat and 1.5 grams of trans fat. There are 1,010 milligrams of sodium and eight grams of sugar.

Luckily, many fast food restaurants have recently added salads to their menu. These are generally low in fat and sodium. Some contain nutritious foods such as mixed greens, vegetables, and lean chicken. Yogurt is another healthy choice, better than the dairy freeze ice cream cone. If you're in a hurry and hit the greasy spoon, here's my suggestion: Grab a salad, especially one loaded with vegetables and lean white chicken, a fruit and yogurt parfait, a courtesy cup of water, and leave.

Better yet, if you have a few minutes, make your own fast food at home. Try a vegetarian garden burger with a whole grain bun. Accompany it with a salad loaded with vegetables. Use vinegar and a little olive oil or a light salad dressing. For dessert, have low-fat yogurt, preferably with fresh fruit.

This healthy, home-made meal will take little time to prepare. Or, would you prefer to drive to a burger joint, wait in line behind five other cars, give your order, wait again, pay, wait again, get poor food, then drive somewhere else to eat?

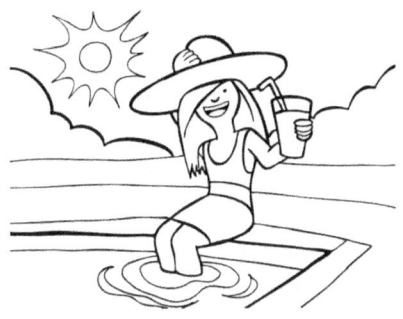

Chapter Five – Individual Food Groups

Many readers may have no idea what to eat from individual food groups. In this chapter, we'll go into greater detail about several food groups including two of the most controversial, meat and dairy products. Should you eliminate meat completely? What if you do and feel less energy? Will you lack any important nutrients? What about milk and dairy products? Should you avoid milk altogether? And, if you do, what nutrients will you lack? Only calcium? Or does milk contain other essential nutrients not easily found in the diet? One nutritionist praises the protein content of meat while another recommends eating no meat. One researcher touts the calcium content of milk and its benefit in preventing osteoporosis while another states flatly that human beings should not consume cow's milk. How does an intelligent person choose?

Let's dive into these areas fearlessly.

Meat

Meat contains lots of important nutrients, such as zinc, iron, phosphorous, selenium, niacin, a small amount of calcium, and the important Vitamin B_{12}. Pork contains Vitamin D. Meat contains lots of protein. Many types of meat are high in saturated fat but contain minimal carbohydrate and no sugar or fiber.

Research shows that vegetarians have a lower risk of certain types of cancer, heart disease, high blood pressure, diabetes, obesity, and gout. Recent research emphasizes eating more fruits, vegetables, whole grains, and less meat.

Meat has a growing number of critics. Many farms feed their cattle growth hormones, steroids, and antibiotics. Several organizations criticize the treatment of animals that aren't allowed to roam the pasture but are kept in cramped cages under unsanitary conditions. Other critics point out the high saturated fat content of meat. Organ meats, such as liver, kidney, and brain, are particularly high in saturated fat.

Should we rid our diets of meat completely? For some people, the answer is yes, but this doesn't apply to everyone.

Let's take a look at two vegetarian diets as objectively as possible.

The first is the Ornish diet, popularized by Dr. Dean Ornish. This regimen includes no meat, fish, poultry, or oils. Non-fat dairy products are allowed, which means that patients have a source of calcium and Vitamin D. Research has shown that this diet, coupled with other aspects of the program, including meditation and exercise, can reverse hardening of the arteries. Your doctor may recommend this diet if you have been diagnosed with severe coronary artery disease (narrowing of the arteries in your heart) or if this condition runs in your family.

Many physicians were astounded when studies of patients on this diet actually showed *reversal* of the narrowing of the coronary arteries. For years, conventional thinking was that the process was irreversible without an invasive procedure such as angioplasty or open heart surgery. (In *angioplasty*, a small balloon at the end of a fine wire catheter is threaded into the coronary arteries and inflated to dilate the effected segments. During *open heart surgery*, the surgeon takes blood vessels harvested from the patient's own calves and grafts them onto the heart to provide extra blood supply.) Incredibly, the arteries of patients on the Ornish diet opened up and transported more blood without mechanical intervention such as dilation or surgery. Some debate remains as to which of these three interventions, diet, meditation, or exercise, is most instrumental in dilating the arteries. Certainly, all three are helpful.

Thus, the Ornish Diet is great news for people who already have hardening of the arteries but want to avoid surgery. The diet is also good for those patients who have a family history of hardening of the arteries, especially heart attacks or strokes, but have not yet developed a problem themselves.

The downside is that this is a fairly restrictive diet and may be hard for some people to follow. Many of my patients love a burger, especially one loaded with extras like cheese, bacon, and mayonnaise, all high in saturated fat. Others salivate at the thought of a juicy steak. However, even those who have no family or personal history of stroke or heart attack can benefit from eating more fruits, vegetables, and whole grains.

This diet allows non-fat dairy products, such as skim milk. Therefore, patients have a source of those nutrients most elusive to vegetarians, calcium, Vitamin D, and Vitamin B_{12}.

The *vegan* diet is even stricter, since it allows no animal products such as eggs and dairy products (milk, cream, butter, and yogurt). This diet can be low in saturated fat and high in vitamins, minerals, and fiber. Since vegetarians still need considerable calories to run the metabolic processes of their bodies, these calories must be obtained from foods other than meat.

If the calories come from fruits, vegetables, seeds, nuts, and beans, then the diet can remain healthy. Unfortunately, many patients in the US tend to substitute cake, candy, cookies, donuts, and soda pop for the lost calories from meat, eggs, and dairy. Such a trade off isn't necessarily healthy, and certainly not similar to the vegan diet in a country like India, where processed foods aren't consumed to the same degree.

An extremely restrictive diet such as a vegan diet may not be best for everyone, for two reasons:

First, the more limited your diet, the greater the risk of a deficiency of some essential nutrient, not only Vitamin B_{12} but also calcium and Vitamin D, both of which are vital for bone construction. Someone who eats a vegan diet with no dairy products or eggs must obtain these nutrients elsewhere. We'll take an extensive look at calcium and Vitamin D in the next section on dairy products and eggs.

Contrary to the claims of some vegetarians, research shows that Vitamin B_{12} is only found in meat sources. There are no vegetables that contain Vitamin B_{12}. Fermented soy products, tempeh, algae, and sea vegetables contain B_{12} analogues, which are not bioavailable to human beings. Luckily, the body can store B_{12}, a water-soluble vitamin, for months or years.

Second, there is a considerable pool of research showing significant benefits from the foods left out of a strict vegetarian diet. For example, several studies show that people who eat fish live longer than people who don't. This advantage may be due to the omega-3 fatty acids contained in fish. Recent studies have also shown that people suffering from depression benefit from the omega-3 fatty acids contained in fish.

What do I recommend for meat lovers? Don't eat the "ugly meats" listed in Chapter Four, mostly derived from pork, that are high in saturated fat, calories, and nitrites: bacon, pepperoni, sausage, bologna, salami, and hot dogs. Bacon, sausage, and pepperoni are high in the proportion of calories derived from fat compared to protein, in a 3:1 ratio. Shy away from beef that's high in saturated fat, such as ground beef, ribs, prime rib, and pot roast. The red meat you eat should be lean, containing relatively little fat. Many super markets carry ground beef that's ninety-three percent lean. Suctioning off the grease after cooking will further lower the saturated fat content. If you're at a restaurant, choose filet mignon, which is quite lean, and avoid prime rib, which is marbled with fat.

Chicken and turkey are leaner meats. They contain approximately half saturated and half unsaturated fat. White meat contains roughly half the fat found in dark meat. So, if you remove the skin, trim off all visible fat, and choose white meat instead of dark, you can remove three-quarters of the fat content of poultry while retaining its nutrients.

People who like to experiment can include other lean meats such as buffalo, antelope, rabbit, and deer. (If you like mnemonics, the first letters of these four animals spell "BARD," although I'm relatively sure that Shakespeare did not eat much buffalo or antelope).

Baked or broiled meat contains less fat than fried. Contrary to popular belief, frying unhealthy meat doesn't make it much healthier. For example, frying bacon drops the fat content of a one hundred gram serving from forty-five grams to forty-one grams, not a great difference. The cholesterol per serving is slightly higher, since red meat contains more cholesterol than the lard that is fried off. Whenever possible, bake or broil your poultry and fish. Don't eat red meat more than three times a week, even if it's low fat. You will derive benefit from eating less red meat and more fruits, vegetables, and whole grains, even if you have great coronary arteries.

Observe how you *feel* on your chosen diet. Some people try a vegetarian diet and don't feel well due to a lack of stamina. Mark Allen was an incredible six-time winner of the grueling Ironman Triathlon, which includes swimming two miles, running twenty-six miles, and bicycling one hundred miles. He was a vegetarian for years, but found that he lacked the endurance and stamina he needed. After putting meat back into his diet, his endurance and stamina promptly improved. Ultimately, diet is a personal choice. Eating healthily means eating what makes you feel strong and well.

Experiment with different *healthy* diets and see how you feel. Keep other variables, such as exercise and sleep, unchanged during your experiment, so that if you do feel different, you can attribute this to the diet, not to other variables. Of course, it's best to get adequate sleep and to exercise regularly, so hopefully you have instituted these changes when you begin to experiment with different diets. Be cautious of any diet that *completely* eliminates any food group, such as fruits, vegetables, grains, meats, or dairy products. You can read more in the chapter entitled "Evaluating Other Diets."

You are the boss. You will decide what you eat. Here are my recommendations:

My personal advice is that the healthiest diet is largely plant-based or "near vegetarian," but may contain a small portion of lean meat once a day or, better yet, two to three times a week. A great way to cut meat from your diet is to avoid meat for breakfast and lunch. The breakfast meats, bacon, sausage, and ham, and luncheon meats, such as bologna and salami, are particularly high in saturated fat and are cured with nitrites. Why not skip meat for breakfast and lunch? For dinner, you can substitute beans or fish for meat several times a week. They provide an excellent protein replacement for meat. If you still have low energy, add a small amount of lean meat. Pay attention to how you feel after the changes.

You can find a table of meats with all of the nutrients listed in Appendix C.

Dairy Products, Eggs, Calcium, Vitamin D, and Sunlight

Dairy products, which include milk, cheese, yogurt, and butter, have also become controversial. Some researchers proclaim that cow's milk is only for suckling calves. Others state emphatically that we shouldn't eat any dairy products at all. Yet many nutritionists drink milk and consume dairy products and tout the value of various dairy products, especially yogurt.

Whole milk contains carbohydrate, protein, and fat in almost equal amounts. Skim milk contains almost no fat. Milk also contains phosphorous, magnesium, potassium, and small amounts of virtually every necessary nutrient including folate and Vitamin K. No wonder many nutritionists tout the value of milk.

Ice cream has a similar profile to milk but contains more fat. Butter is highest in total fat and saturated fat. Butter contains fewer nutrients than milk except for large amounts of Vitamin A.

There are three ingredients in milk that people may have trouble digesting. First, some people are lactose intolerant and have trouble digesting lactose, the sugar in milk. Second, others cannot digest casein, the protein in milk. Third, still others have trouble digesting the fat in milk, especially in whole milk or cream.

In my medical practice, I've noticed that the vast majority of people can and do consume dairy products without a problem. Even patients who are diagnosed as lactose intolerant can again become able to digest lactose simply by adding a small amount of milk to their diet and gradually increasing that amount daily within their comfort level. If they experience abdominal cramping or diarrhea, they temporarily decrease the amount of milk they consume. Some patients have more difficulty with the fat content than the lactose, so drinking skim milk makes digestion easier. The following table shows the relative calorie, fat, and protein content of whole and skim milk:

	Calories	Protein, grams	Fat, grams
1 cup whole milk	160	9	9
1 cup skim milk	90	9	Trace

Yogurt is often well tolerated, in patients who have trouble with milk. Yogurt contains live and active yogurt cultures, which may aid in digestion and in the bacterial balance of the intestinal tract. Most yogurt has no added Vitamin D.

Most adult bone mass is laid down during the second decade of life, from age ten to twenty. Consistent milk consumption during this age increases bone density, which may guard against osteoporosis later. People who do *not* eat dairy products have a difficult time getting sufficient calcium in their diet. While other foods contain calcium, none provide the amount that milk and dairy products do. Low-fat dairy products, such as skim milk, 1% milk, and yogurt, are a rich source of calcium while remaining low in fat.

Any food that can provide the total nutrition for a growing calf has to be packed with nutrients. An eight ounce glass of 1% milk contains the following:

NUTRIENT	AMOUNT PER 8 OUNCES 1% MILK	% RDA
Calcium	250 mg	25
Vitamin B$_{12}$	1.0 mcg	33
Magnesium	25 mg	6
Riboflavin	0.425 mg	25
Potassium	274 mg	8
Zinc	2.0 mg	16
Vitamin A	450 IU	9
Vitamin D	120 IU	30

Note that the manufacturer adds the last two ingredients.

What do I recommend? Milk is a nutritious food. Unless you have trouble with digestion, consuming some dairy products is a good idea. Emphasize the low-fat variety such as skim milk and yogurt. Infants from birth to age one are healthiest if breast fed, followed by formula. Infants under one year old should drink *no* cow's milk. They are unable to digest it and may have subsequent intestinal bleeding. Children from one to two years of age can drink 2% milk since their high metabolism and growth rate utilize the extra calories and fat. At age two, most pediatricians recommend switching to 1% milk. If you're in doubt about milk, talk to your doctor or a nutritionist.

If you have trouble digesting milk but need it as a calcium source, try yogurt with Vitamin D added or as a supplement. If you can't digest milk products and are allergic to soy, choose healthy servings of the other calcium-rich foods listed below.

Eggs are another controversial food due to the high cholesterol content. They aren't a dairy product since they're not derived from milk. However, since they are one of the rare foods that contain natural calcium and Vitamin D, this is a good time to consider them.

Eggs are a spectacularly nutritious food. High in protein, they're a good source of calcium, phosphorous, potassium, iron, selenium, folate, Vitamin A, Vitamin D, and zinc. All the cholesterol and many of the nutrients in the egg are in the yolk. Two large eggs contain 1.3 mcg of the elusive Vitamin B_{12} (the recommended amount is 2.4 mcg daily). No wonder they've been called a nutrition powerhouse.

Dieticians generally allow two medium eggs twice a week for most patients, with the exception of those who have coronary artery disease or who have been advised to avoid eggs by their doctor. Of course, if you are allergic to eggs, you shouldn't eat them. Each yolk contains approximately 250 milligrams of cholesterol. Egg white contains no cholesterol. Many low cholesterol diets use egg whites instead of the whole egg.

You need 1,000 milligrams of calcium daily (1,200 if you're over fifty). Eight ounces of milk or yogurt contains about 250 milligrams of calcium. So, you need approximately three servings daily to provide a total of 750 milligrams of calcium, since you will derive some calcium from other foods. If you choose not to drink milk or can't digest it well, the following foods or supplements are rich in calcium:

NON-DAIRY FOODS RICH IN CALCIUM

1.) Sardines with the bones
2.) Halibut, herring, lobster, shrimp, trout
3.) Soybeans, tofu, or soy milk
4.) Collard greens, turnip greens, kale, broccoli, spinach, okra, beet greens
5.) Most beans, including lentils, kidney beans, white beans
6.) Almonds, hazelnuts, Brazil nuts, some seeds
7.) Calcium carbonate antacid tablets (Tums®)
8.) Calcium plus Vitamin D tablets (Os Cal® and many other brands)
9.) Tahini (sesame paste)
10.) Calcium-fortified juice
11.) Figs
12.) Molasses

However, calcium without Vitamin D is not very helpful in building strong bones. As we see in the Merck table, Vitamin D helps us to absorb calcium in the gut, to implant calcium into bone, and to reabsorb lost calcium through the kidneys.

The current rage in the medical field is evidence-based research. A medical author will gather and evaluate all available studies regarding a specific diagnosis. The effects of various treatments for this diagnosis are rated under the following five categories, in descending order of effectiveness:

1.) Beneficial
2.) Likely to be beneficial
3.) Unknown effectiveness
4.) Unlikely to be beneficial
5.) Likely to be ineffective or harmful

For fracture prevention in post-menopausal women, calcium plus Vitamin D receives the highest rating, beneficial. Calcium alone and Vitamin D alone are each given a poor rating, unlikely to be beneficial. So, we need both Vitamin D and calcium both.

Recent research shows that Vitamin D may have other important properties. These include building muscle mass, preventing periodontal disease, and decreasing the incidence of certain cancers, such as pancreatic cancer.

Unfortunately, Vitamin D can be rather elusive. Here's why.

You can convert the inactive form of Vitamin D to the metabolically active form by getting about twenty to thirty minutes of sunlight daily while not wearing sunscreen. A light-skinned person in the sun in a bathing suit converts about 20,000 international units in a half an hour. Darker-skinned patients convert less but nevertheless make an adequate supply.

The farther you are from the equator, the weaker the sun's rays. If you live in Florida or Mexico, you can convert sunlight year round. If you live north of a line from Atlanta to Los Angeles, the sun's rays are too weak to convert Vitamin D from November through February. If you live in Canada, the sun's rays are too weak from October through March, or for six months of the year. This means that all of your Vitamin D intake must come from food or supplements. But since the angle of the sun limits the amount of UV-B radiation that traverses our atmosphere, your skin can't convert Vitamin D before 8 a.m. or after 5 p.m. any season of the year, including summer.

Are there any people who thrive in a northern climate? Well, yes, the Eskimos do. Their diet is rich in fatty fish. Some fish are high in both calcium and Vitamin D. These include herring, sardines, and shrimp.

If you make a sufficient supply of this fat-soluble vitamin during the summer, you can store it in your fat and use it during winter. However, no one really knows how much we store. It's best to get regular adequate amounts of Vitamin D.

The following foods are rich in natural Vitamin D.

FOOD	Vitamin D, IU
Cat fish, 3 ounces, cooked	570
Sockeye salmon, ¼ cup, canned	480
Pink salmon, ¼ cup, canned	290
Shrimp, 3 ounces, cooked	170
Tuna, light, ¼ cup, canned	130
Egg, 1 medium	20

IU = International Units

The following foods have Vitamin D added by the manufacturer.

FOOD	Vitamin D, IU
Milk, 1 cup	100
Soy milk, 1 cup, most brands	100 – 120
Orange juice, fortified, 1 cup	100

The following table lists the Vitamin D content of various species of fish:

FISH	Vitamin D Content, IU per 7 ounce portion
Herring	3,256
Catfish	1,000
Pacific sardines	960
Atlantic sardines	544
Shrimp	304
Flounder	120
Atlantic cod	88

FISH	Vitamin D Content, IU per 7 ounce portion
Haddock	0
Halibut	0
Lobster	0
Pacific oyster	0
Atlantic salmon	0
Trout	0
Tuna	0

Note that there is a tremendous variation in the amount of Vitamin D contained in different species of fish. Herring provides over 3,000 IU per serving. Several species provide none.

The Institute of Medicine recommends a daily intake of 400 IU of Vitamin D. However, 800 IU daily decreases the incidence of hip fractures while lesser amounts don't. Many nutritionists now state that we should get at least 1,000 IU daily. With the added benefits of Vitamin D that have been documented recently, some nutritionists recommend 2,000 to 4,000 IU daily.

My recommendation is that you should get 1,000 milligrams daily. Only take more than 1,000 milligrams after consulting with your doctor, as there is a slight chance that higher levels of Vitamin D can lead to an increased formation of kidney stones.

There are two ways to get adequate Vitamin D.

First, get twenty minutes of sunlight while not wearing sunscreen and exposing at least your hands, face, and arms between 8 a.m. and 5 p.m. during the sunny seasons of the year.

Second, during late fall and winter in the northern and southern latitudes, drink three cups of skim or 1% milk daily. Eat fish rich in Vitamin D at least twice a week. Or take a daily supplement of 400 milligrams.

Oils

The Mediterranean diet includes lots of olive oil. People prepare food with olive oil and even dip their bread in it. Many live to a ripe old age. Does this mean we should include lots of olive oil in our diet?

Let's look at oils more thoroughly. First, let's have the facts.

ALL oils derive all of their calories from fat. ALL oils contain a mixture of monounsaturated, polyunsaturated, and saturated fat, but in widely varying ratios, with some oils containing mostly monounsaturated fat, some mostly polyunsaturated fat, and some mostly saturated fat.

Oils contain no protein or carbohydrate, including no sugar. They contain no cholesterol and no water. Most oils contain very few nutrients. Plant-derived oils contain vitamins E and K.

Doctors still debate the relative merits or demerits of different oils. Dr. Dean Ornish doesn't recommend it to his patients with narrowing of the coronary arteries. Dr. Andrew Weil, a respected expert in preventive medicine, and Dr. Barry Sears, author of the Zone diet, both feel that olive oil in moderation is a good source of polyunsaturated fat and part of a balanced diet. When the experts argue, what are us small fry to do?

Here are the oils and butters that contain the most saturated fat, with the worst first:

Oils High In Saturated Fat

Coconut oil	Palm oil
Palm kernel oil	Beef tallow
Cocoa butter	Lard
Butter	

Here are the oils that are lowest in saturated fat, with the least saturated fat first:

Oils Low In Saturated Fat

Safflower oil	Olive
Canola	Sesame
Flaxseed	Soybean
Sunflower	Peanut
Corn	

Peanut oil, the highest in saturated fat of the healthy oils, contains less than one quarter of the amount of saturated fat in coconut oil.

Researchers generally rank the healthier oils based on the predominant type of fat that they contain.

Olive, canola, and peanut oil contain monounsaturated fats. Monounsaturated oils may have protective effects on the heart and blood vessels and are considered the healthiest.

Corn, safflower, and fish oil contain mostly polyunsaturated fats. Coconut, palm kernel, and palm oils contain lots of saturated fat, as does lard.

Fish oil is the new favorite on the block but isn't used for cooking or salads.

What do I recommend? My recommendation is that you use canola oil and olive oil about equally and in moderation in preference to other oils. When you use olive oil to prepare food, look for extra-virgin olive oil. Although it's more expensive, as it's derived from the first pressing of olives, it's the least processed. Soybean oil is healthy but already comprises about seventy-five percent of the oil in store-bought foods, such as mayonnaise, salad dressings, and pastries, so you won't need more.

Avoid the saturated oils, namely, palm and coconut oil. Lard, coconut, palm, and palm kernel oils contain mostly saturated fats. *Lard* is hogs' fat melted down into a soft white solid. Any oil that the manufacturer alters, such as hydrogenated oil, also contains trans fats. Look for foods with no lard in the ingredients. Avoid hydrogenated oils.

If we rank the oils, with the "healthier" oils floating to the top, it would look something like this:

Healthier Oils
Canola, olive oil, fish oil - best
Corn, soy, safflower, sesame, soybean, peanut – also good
Coconut, palm, palm kernel oils, lard - bad

Fiber

Let's review some facts about fiber.

Fiber is the indigestible part of plant foods. A high-fiber diet helps control insulin levels, triglycerides, and cholesterol. Patients who eat a high-fiber diet have a lower occurrence of heart attacks, strokes, and diabetes. Fiber helps prevent weight gain by conferring a feeling of fullness without the consumption of high-calorie foods. Fiber aids in the management of diverticulosis, the small pouches frequently seen in the wall of the colon in those over sixty years of age.

Fiber helps in the movement of stool in the colon, reducing transit time. Fiber, along with extra fluids, acts as a natural antidote to constipation. Populations that eat a high fiber diet have a lower incidence of cancer of the colon than those who don't. One reason may be that any carcinogens in the diet have less time in contact with the colon since fiber makes food pass through the colon more quickly. Cultures that eat a lot of fiber avoid processed foods and the million-and-one additives that manufacturers include, which may also be part of the reason for the lower incidence of cancer of the colon.

Studies show a correlation between a high-fiber diet and improvement in blood cholesterol levels, irritable bowel syndrome, Crohn's disease, constipation, hemorrhoids, obesity, and even varicose veins.

There are hundreds of different soluble and insoluble fibers. Each has different physiological effects. Of course, since they include fruits, vegetables, whole grains, peas, and beans, high fiber foods are wonderful for their nutritional content, too. Note that all of these great high-fiber foods are plant-based and unprocessed. Specifically, soluble fiber is found in oats, barley, legumes, and citrus fruits. Insoluble fiber is found in wheat bran and vegetables. Although there is individual variation, beans and lentils have the highest amount of fiber per serving of any food group. (Beans again present themselves as an excellent choice of food.)

Meat contains no fiber. Processed grains, such as white flour, have most of the fiber removed.

Miracle Foods

In the course of my research for this chapter, I have accumulated numerous articles trumpeting the virtues of some nutritionist's favorite food. One wrote admiringly of the virtues of winter squash, stating that winter squash contains Vitamin C, potassium, iron, beta carotene, and calcium, with the added benefit of fiber, all at a "cost" of only eighty calories. The author himself eats squash several times a week and feels that it's a key to good health.

Another wrote lovingly of blueberries because of their high content of anti-oxidants, compounds renowned for their ability to neutralize the free radicals that clog arteries and cause cancer. He recommends eating large quantities of blueberries.

Several authors wrote glowing articles promoting the benefits of broccoli, not only as a great cancer fighter, but also as a low calorie, high fiber, vitamin rich food. One nutritionist wrote an article about "great greens" and recommended chard, bok choy, spinach, and collards, among others. In yet another article, the author praises dandelion, watercress, endive, kale, and chicory. Most of us have heard that "an apple a day keeps the doctor away." Apples contain quercetin, which some nutritionists claim can alleviate diabetes and asthma and possibly decrease the incidence of lung cancer.

Dr. Weil, the Harvard-trained medical doctor and leading expert in the field of complementary and alternative medicine, extols the virtues of garlic. He calls garlic a superior tonic for the heart and blood vessels, stating that it lowers blood pressure, reduces total cholesterol, raises levels of HDL (the good cholesterol), and inhibits blood clotting. He also feels that garlic may serve as an anti-cancer agent and a natural antibiotic.

What are we to make of these claims by doctors or nutritionists regarding the wonderful characteristics of a single food? What has research confirmed?

Several studies have found that people who eat more fruits and vegetables have a lower incidence of cancer of the stomach, esophagus, mouth, lung, and colon. Nutritionists now recommend eight to ten servings of fruit and vegetables a day instead of the previously recommended five, and several servings of whole grains daily.

As noted, however, the research is far from perfect. It's difficult to isolate the benefits of a single food while attempting to control for all of the other variables of human health.

All of these foods - squash, blueberries, broccoli, garlic, and the various greens such as bok choy and Swiss chard - contain dynamic compounds that may prolong life and help to fight disease. Although every researcher and nutritionist seems to have a favorite food, it is doubtful that consuming any *one* of them in large quantities will allow you to live to the age of Methuselah. We must exert caution when recommending foods as preventive options for specific disease.

There is no perfect food. The excessive consumption of one item at the expense of others leads to a limited intake of potentially beneficial compounds, some of which haven't been discovered yet. While some compounds in these foods are extremely helpful, it's unlikely that medical research will find a single ingredient that acts like a magic bullet to prevent cancer, diabetes, or other diseases.

I recommend each of these foods heartily as part of an overall healthy diet and lifestyle, but can't attribute miraculous properties to any of them. What does perform miracles is eating a healthy, balanced diet, meal after meal, day after day. Include your favorite food often, if you wish, but not to the exclusion of the other healthy foods. Each fruit, vegetable, bean, nut, and grain, in its own unique way, adds a combination of nutrients to our bodies. A key recommendation is to vary your diet, including as many of these healthy foods as possible, in reasonable quantities.

One study showed that the average American consumes only fifteen different foods each week. If we eat only the same three vegetables, such as carrots, celery, and cauliflower, every day, we miss a lot. The same is true of eating only bananas, oranges, and apples for fruits. Look for fruits and vegetables that you don't eat often. Add them to your grocery cart.

Eat a wide variety of healthy foods. Not only is this good sense, but more fun. Some unusual fruits you may want to try are papaya, mango, kiwi, apricots, and even prunes (no, prunes are not just for the elderly, but they do help patients with constipation). You can also buy juices made from virtually every fruit and some vegetables. Indulge yourself in the pleasure of trying vegetables such as Swiss chard, bok choy, endive, dandelions, and kale. Try a slice of avocado as an unusual addition to your sandwich.

Why not try one or two healthy new foods this week? Add a few to your grocery list. You may be deliciously surprised by your experiments.

Let's take a look at a table of these miracle ingredients and their food sources, along with their reputed benefits.

MIRACLE INGREDIENT	FOOD SOURCES	REPUTED BENEFITS
Allicin	Garlic, onions, leeks	Decreased coronary artery disease, cancer prevention
Anthocyanins	Blueberries, strawberries	Prevent arteriosclerosis, cancer
Carotenoids (lutein, lycopene, others)	Colorful fruits and vegetables	Decreased cataracts, macular degeneration, arteriosclerosis, some cancers

MIRACLE INGREDIENT	FOOD SOURCES	REPUTED BENEFITS
Isothiocyanates	Cruciferous vegetables	Slow breast cancer growth in animals
Indoles	Cruciferous vegetables	Slow breast cancer growth in animals
Mono unsaturated fatty acids, polyphenols	Olive oil	Clean coronary arteries, decrease blood pressure
Omega-3 fatty acids	Salmon, sardines, mackerel, herring, walnuts, flax seed, canola oil	Reduced heart attack, stroke, macular degeneration, various cancers
Phytoestrogens, isoflavones	Soy nuts	Decrease blood pressure, hot flashes in post-menopausal women
Polyphenols	Green, red, black teas	Anti-oxidants inactivate cell-damaging free radicals. Prevent blood clotting, lower cholesterol, prevent arthritis.
Quercetin	Apples, broccoli, citrus fruits	Reduce arteriosclerosis, inhibit cancer cells, preserve vision
Soluble fiber Insoluble fiber	Some fruits and vegetables, barley, oats, beans Some fruits and vegetables, almonds, barley, brown rice, whole wheat	Decrease serum cholesterol, reduced coronary artery disease Decrease constipation, hemorrhoids, diverticulits, possible colon cancer
Terpenes	Citrus fruits	Reduce risk of cancer

Note that *cruciferous* vegetables derive their name from the Latin word crux for cross which refers to the shape of the blossoms. These plants in the mustard family include broccoli, cauliflower, Brussels sprouts, kale, rutabaga, turnips, and mustard seed.

These miracle ingredients are mainly found in fruits and vegetables, occasionally in a whole grain, oil, or fish. None of them are found in meat.

Take a good look at the middle column. Note that many of these are the "Good Foods" from the list of "The Good, the Bad, and the

Ugly." We have more reassuring evidence that our diet recommendations are right on the mark.

Great Foods from Individual Food Groups

Over the years, I've collected lists with titles like "The Top 100 Foods" or "The Ten Healthiest Vegetables." The following sections will give you some idea of what foods are most often recommended by the experts. Some of them are common in restaurants; most can be found in the grocery store. This is not all-inclusive, so please don't limit yourself. Experiment.

You can find extensive tables of the nutrients in these foods in Appendix C.

Great Vegetables

Vegetables are a great addition to the diet. They contain no cholesterol. Except for the avocado, none contain any significant amount of fat. They are low in calories and sodium. Most are high in fiber, folic acid, and potassium. The dark green, yellow, or orange vegetables contain Vitamin A or its precursor, carotene. Vegetables with dark green leaves usually contain iron and riboflavin. Virtually every vegetable contains some Vitamin C. Traditionally many cultures around the world eat vegetables with every meal except breakfast.

Vegetables are especially important to the diabetic diet. They don't cause a prompt rise in insulin and blood sugar levels. They are extremely low in calories. Indeed, one-half cup of most vegetables contains about fifty calories. Even the "starchy" vegetables such as peas, corn, lima beans, and white potatoes contain only fifty to one hundred calories in a half a cup.

When diabetic patients eat more vegetables and whole grains instead of their usual staple of junk food and refined flour, their blood sugar levels drop, their insulin requirements fall, they feel better, and they have more energy. The difference in how they feel can be incredible. As one patient told me, "If I had known that I would feel this much better after changing my diet, I would have done it twenty years ago."

Any veggies are better than none at all. However, if you have the opportunity, choose fresh before frozen and frozen before canned.

Always choose unsalted vegetables, if possible; otherwise, rinse the salted vegetables before eating. I'll have more to say about purchasing vegetables in a later chapter.

Deeply colored vegetables usually have more vitamins and minerals than their lighter cousins. The government actually divides vegetables into five groups and recommends eating vegetables from each group every week. These groups are:

1.) Orange vegetables, including carrots, sweet potatoes, pumpkin, and winter squash;
2.) Green vegetables, including broccoli, spinach, kale, collards, and turnip greens;
3.) Legumes, or beans, including chick peas and tofu;
4.) Starchy vegetables, including corn, white potatoes, and green peas; and,
5.) Other vegetables, a miscellaneous category including just about everything else.

The best advice is to eat a wide variety of different vegetables. Don't just serve one vegetable with your meal. Serve a vegetable medley. Supermarkets now carry packs of frozen vegetables that contain up to ten varieties per bag. You can microwave these vegetables in seconds. Eat a rainbow of vegetables, including some orange, red, yellow, purple, dark green, leafy green, and white. The rainbow on your plate is not only beautiful to look at but has beautiful effects inside your body.

Iceberg lettuce is mostly water and contains minimal calories and minimal nutrients. Better choices of lettuce include romaine, red leaf, and bib lettuce, which are easily accessible in the grocery store. Turnip or collard greens are also healthy, but should be cooked with onions, green pepper, or other vegetables, not with salt pork, bacon, or ham hocks. For the ambitious, bok choy and Swiss chard are great choices and can be stir fried with a small amount of healthy oil.

The following "great vegetables" contain varying amounts of potassium, iron, folate, Vitamin C, Vitamin K, carotenoids, fiber. *Carotenoids* are red or yellow pigments in plants that the body converts to Vitamin A. The first three powerhouse vegetables contain all seven of these nutrients. The first seven in the list all contain healthy amounts of Vitamin K.

GREAT VEGETABLES

1.) Spinach
2.) Collard greens
3.) Brussel sprouts
4.) Swiss chard
5.) Kale
6.) Pumpkin
7.) Broccoli
8.) Sweet potato
9.) Carrots
10.) Endive
11.) Red, yellow pepper
12.) Butternut squash
13.) Romaine lettuce
14.) Asparagus
15.) Peas
16.) Okra
17.) Zucchini
18.) Acorn squash
19.) Cauliflower
20.) Corn
21.) Green pepper
22.) Green beans

Some vegetables have few of the above nutrients. They include the following:

VEGETABLES THAT ARE NUTRIENT-POOR

Alfalfa sprouts
Eggplant
Cucumber
Garlic
Radishes
Turnips
Onions
Celery

Should you skip these vegetables? No. Garlic and onions contain allium and flavonoids, which are postulated to prevent cancer. Celery has few nutrients but does have Vitamin K. Some vegetables may contain helpful compounds which science simply hasn't recognized yet. Cook with garlic and onions but emphasize the other vegetables in your daily diet.

Again, eat a wide variety of vegetables.

You'll find three tables of great vegetables and their nutrient content in Appendix C.

Great Fruits

Fruits are another vital component of a healthy diet. Fruits contain no cholesterol and only a tiny amount of saturated fat. They contain minimal protein. They are high in carbohydrate, one-half to two-thirds of which is sugar. This varies greatly among the individual fruits. Grapes contain fifteen times as much total sugar as rhubarb, which contains a very low 1.1 grams per one hundred grams. Apples, bananas, cherries, and mangoes all contain more than ten grams of sugar per one hundred grams of edible fruit. The fruits that are lowest in sugar content are rhubarb, blackberries, raspberries, and strawberries.

Fruits are a good source of Vitamin A, Vitamin C, and potassium. Some of the orange fruits in particular, such as apricots, cantaloupe, mango, and peaches, contain a significant amount of Vitamin A, but so do plums and watermelon. Fruits contain minimal iron and no Vitamin B_{12}.

Fruits are rich in fiber. Blackberries, guava, and raspberries all contain more than five grams of fiber per one hundred gram serving.

Many nutritionists have their favorite lists of great fruits. Here are some excellent choices that are rich in nutrients, particularly Vitamin C, potassium, and carotenoids. Except for cantaloupe and honeydew, these fruits contain significant amounts of fiber.

GREAT FRUITS

1.) Papaya
2.) Guava
3.) Watermelon
4.) Grapefruit (red or pink have more nutrients than white)
5.) Cantaloupe
6.) Kiwi
7.) Apricots
8.) Oranges
9.) Strawberries
10.) Blackberries
11.) Raspberries
12.) Blueberries
13.) Peaches
14.) Mango
15.) Honeydew

Some fruits and fruit products are not particularly nutritious. They include the following:

MEDIOCRE FRUITS AND FRUIT PRODUCTS

Apple sauce
Cranberry sauce
Fruit cocktail
Canned peaches, pears, pineapple
Dried prunes
Raisins
Some common fruits, such as bananas and apples, hit the middle

tier. Although they don't contain as many nutrients as our first choices, they are still healthy. Apples contain quercetin, which, as we've seen, some nutritionists consider a miracle ingredient.

You'll find three tables of great fruits and their nutrient content in Appendix C.

Great Beans

Beans are good source of carbohydrate and protein. They contain little fat, except for garbanzo and soy beans, which contain modest amounts of unsaturated fat. They contain no cholesterol. They are an excellent source of fiber, except for soybeans, which contain a more modest amount.

Beans are an excellent source of many nutrients, including iron, magnesium, phosphorous, potassium, zinc, manganese, selenium, and niacin. Some contain small amounts of vitamins A and K. Beans make a good substitute for meat for those who wish to decrease their meat consumption. Like fruits, vegetables, oils, and nuts, they contain no Vitamin $B_{12,}$ which, as we now know, is not found in a vegetarian diet.

Beans are an excellent addition to the meal plan. Here are some great choices for beans:

1.) Black
2.) Garbanzo (chick peas)
3.) Kidney
4.) Lentils
5.) Navy
6.) Pinto
7.) Soy
8.) White

You'll find a table of these eight great beans and their nutrient content in Appendix C.

Great Grains

Grains are a good source of protein and carbohydrate, very little of which is sugar. Grains are low in fat, especially saturated fat. They contain no cholesterol.

Grains are a good source of many nutrients, including iron, magnesium, phosphorous, potassium, zinc, manganese, selenium, and niacin. They contain modest amounts of calcium. Some have a small amount of vitamins A and K. Like fruits, vegetables, oils, nuts, and beans, they contain no Vitamin B_{12}.

When choosing foods that contain grains, look for the best – whole grains. Try to avoid processed grains, which have lost much of their fiber and vitamins. When reading the label on bread or pasta, look for a whole grain as the *first* ingredient listed. Some great grains that are easy to find in American grocery stores are:

1.) Oats, oatmeal
2.) Wild or brown rice
3.) Whole wheat or buckwheat
4.) Barley

Unfortunately, for those whose diet consists mainly of "meat and potatoes" and those who love French fries, potatoes don't make the list of great grains. They contain less nutrients and fiber than other grains. Chemical sprays are often used on commercial potatoes. You can decrease the chemical spray content by peeling the potato, but then you lose the fiber. If you eat potatoes, look for the organic variety. They are a good source of fiber (the skin), vitamin B-6, Vitamin C, and potassium.

Why not substitute a sweet potato instead, a healthier alternative? Yams are a variety of sweet potato but contain less beta carotene. These have a thick skin that is protective and is peeled before eating.

Some instant breakfast cereals contain only whole oats. Others, such as Quaker Multi Grain®, contain four whole grains: barley, rye, oats, and wheat. You can remember them by the mnemonic BROW. They cook in two minutes in the microwave.

Luckily, every month there are more choices of cereal on the grocery shelves. Some cereal manufacturers are now formulating their products so that all of their cereals contain whole grains, some with very little sugar and no artificial colors or preservatives. Some even contain only organic whole grains. These are far healthier alternatives to the old days when the two main ingredients of breakfast cereals were sugar and bleached flour.

Corn is also a whole grain. As noted previously, yellow corn is rich in carotenoids, including zeaxanthin and lutein, which the latest research shows may help preserve eyesight. Popcorn made from yellow corn also contains these nutrients. White corn cannot make the same claim. Again, choose the more deeply colored variety. In this case, prefer yellow corn.

Some healthy grains that may be harder to find are:

1.) Quinoa
2.) Bulgur
3.) Millet.

Why not give some of the more unusual varieties a try?

You'll find a table of great grains along with their respective nutrient content in Appendix C.

Great Seafood

Seafood is a great source of protein. Most seafood, except for oysters, contains no carbohydrate. Seafood is low in fat, except for certain species, such as herring and sardines, and low in cholesterol. Seafood contains no fiber. Remember that fish contain the two Omega-3 fatty acids that stabilize heart cells and may allow the heart to maintain a regular heartbeat, thereby decreasing the chances of sudden death.

Fish are a good source of Vitamin B_{12}, especially herring and oysters. Oysters are also rich in zinc, which may endow them with their purported aphrodisiac qualities. Some species of seafood contain both calcium and Vitamin D, such as herring, sardines, and shrimp. You may have noted that the elusive Vitamin D tends to be found in fatty foods, such as fish, like herring and sardines, and in pork.

The following fish are highest in Omega-3 fatty acids, from most to least.

Salmon, wild or coho
Rainbow trout (freshwater)
Herring
Sardines

All of these choices are also low in mercury content, making them great choices. Trout, herring, and sardines also contain significant Vitamin D, making them all around winners.

Swordfish and mackerel contain Omega-3 but have been omitted from the list because of government warnings about high mercury content.

The following fish contain less Omega-3 fatty acids.

Pollock	Cod
Flounder	Crab
Sole	Haddock
Whiting	Catfish
Halibut	Shrimp
Tuna	Clams
Perch	Lobster

Shrimp contains about 200 mg of cholesterol per four ounces, more than any shellfish except squid.

The fish that are highest in mercury are the following:

1.) Shark
2.) Swordfish
3.) King mackerel
4.) Tilefish
5.) Certain tuna, including albacore (white), yellow fin, and tuna steak.

Pregnant women, nursing mothers, and children should avoid these fish completely.

Note that the bigger species of tuna contain more mercury than the smaller species. That's because the bigger fish have eaten more small fish. Albacore tuna can contain up to four times as much mercury as chunk light tuna.

The commercial fish that are lowest in mercury content are the following:

Anchovies	Oyster	Tilapia
Catfish	Perch	Trout
Clams	Pollock	(freshwater)
Cod	Sardine	Tuna (light,
Flounder	Scallops	canned)
Haddock	Shrimp	Whitefish
Herring	Sole	

Many nutrition experts have criticized the government for not keep this information current and making it more available to the public. Pregnant women and children especially need to be careful of the mercury content of fish. My recommendation is that you subscribe to a good newsletter such as the Nutrition Action Health Letter or the Berkeley Wellness Letter.

There are also several helpful websites. One favorite is www.got-mercury.org, run by the non-profit Take Action. They have listed a fun and easy "Mercury Calculator" on the home page. If you eat more than one type of fish per week, one click takes you to their "Advanced Calculator." Calculations take only a few seconds to complete. You get a prompt answer to your mercury consumption based on your weight and the type and amount of fish eaten per week.

The United States Food and Drug Administration's Center for Food Safety and Applied Nutrition lists mercury content at www.cfsan.fda.gov/%7Efrf/sea-mehg.html. You may also call 1-888-SAFE-FOOD for information. Unfortunately, some of the reports cited are as old as 1978. The Environmental Protection Agency sponsors a website, www.epa.gov/waterscience/fish/states.htm. A simple click will transport you to your state's EPA website which contains advice on what specific types of fish to avoid from particular bodies of water in your state.

The following are good choices for seafood, best choices first:

1.) Salmon (Wild is preferable. All Alaskan and most canned salmon is wild.)
2.) Flounder
3.) Sole
4.) Rainbow trout
5.) Haddock
6.) Cod
7.) Halibut (prefer Pacific)
8.) Ocean perch
9.) Pollock
10.) Herring
11.) Tilapia
12.) Mahi mahi
13.) Sardines
14.) Tuna (chunk light preferred to albacore)
15.) Oysters
16.) King crab
17.) Clams
18.) Shrimp.

My recommendation is that you eat a four to six ounce serving of fish three times a week, choosing from a variety of fish on this list.

Ongoing research concerning the benefits of taking fish oil supplements is encouraging. Many nutritionists prefer the fish itself to the oil capsules. When you eat the fish itself, remember to peel the skin from the fish and discard it.

Keep abreast of any developments in the field of nutrition, including the value of various types of fish, their mercury content, and the debate over fish oil supplements.

You'll find two tables of great seafood and the nutrient content in Appendix C.

How to Fill Your Plate

You are now knowledgeable concerning the benefits and drawbacks of an amazing variety of food. You know to eat a balanced diet containing 50% carbohydrates, 30% protein, and 20% fat. While this sounds easy, most patients are confused when it comes to filling their plate according to these guidelines. Here's a simple solution that nutritionists recommend:

Picture a round plate. Divide the plate into four imaginary quarters.

Cover one quarter of the plate with meat or fish, about four ounces.

Cover one quarter of the plate with a healthy starch, such as yams, sweet potatoes, acorn or butternut squash, whole grain brown rice, barley, or occasionally a "starchy" vegetable such as peas, corn, or lima beans.

Cover one-half of the plate with non-starchy vegetables or a salad made from a variety of vegetables and healthy greens. Use a small amount of olive oil.

Place two items outside the plate, your fruit cup and a beverage.

In Appendix A you'll find a simple sample meal plan, which will help you determine great selections for each meal in the proper proportions.

You'll learn more about beverage choices in Chapter Six on Water and Fluids.

Substitutions

So, you've decided to give up most of the ugly foods. Well, what do you eat in their place?

There's lots of room for individual variation on this. Here are some of the most popular foods to cut from the diet and some suggestions for substitutions:

1.) Meat – The top seven foods on the ugly list are fatty meats that have been cured with nitrites. Why not substitute beans for meat? Beans are high in protein and a nutritional powerhouse. They are easy to prepare, inexpensive, and found everywhere.

   Three times a week, substitute fish, a popular item in many diets including the Mediterranean and Japanese diets. Two to three times a week, eat fish, a healthy starch, and a salad or vegetable medley containing at least five to ten fresh vegetables.

   Instead of your bacon double cheese burger, try a soy burger. These are made mainly from soybeans or vegetables. Although the flavor is a little unusual at first, most people develop a taste for them quickly. If your fast food joint doesn't carry garden burgers, try a big salad or a baked chicken sandwich.

   Instead of lunch meat, why not try a vegetarian sandwich? Try a tofu, tomato, and avocado sandwich. You can add a variety of greens like endive or Swiss chard, some onion, or even garlic to your sandwich. How about mushroom, eggplant, and avocado on whole grain bread? Here your creativity can really flourish.

2.) Soda – Many of my patients consume great quantities of soda, which we in the Midwest call pop. One patient mentioned that he drank seventeen cans of a cola drink daily; another young woman drank at least two two-liter bottles of soda a day. Not surprisingly, these patients often present to the doctor with fatigue or no energy. They have substituted the empty calories in soda for the far better fuel sources found in a balanced diet.

Why not substitute fruits or fruit juices? They will satisfy your energy and fluid needs in a much healthier fashion. In addition to a refreshing and delicious taste, they provide vitamins, minerals, and fiber.

If you're still thirsty, or if you're diabetic, Mother Nature's best drink for satisfying a fluid deficit is water. Yes, water. There are no calories, sugar, fat, salt, or cholesterol in water. Herbal tea is another good substitute. Green and black teas contain caffeine so drink these in moderation.

3.) Snacks – Many people grab a candy bar, cookies, potato chips, or a doughnut for a snack. These are made from refined white flour, are high in sugar, salt, calories, fat, and sometimes cholesterol, and are often loaded with artificial colors, flavors, and preservatives.

Instead, air-popped, unsalted, and unbuttered yellow popcorn makes a great snack. For convenience, it is hard to beat microwave popcorn. Choose a variety that's low in salt and fat.

Fresh fruit makes a quick and healthy snack. Vegetables are also excellent snacks, easy to pack, and nice to nibble on as finger foods. Nuts contain more fat but are rich in unsaturated fats, including monounsaturated fats, as well as fiber, Vitamin E, folic acid, and other B vitamins. Some nuts, like almonds, contain calcium. The omega-3 fatty acids in walnuts are quite heart smart. Grab a handful of almonds and walnuts for your snack.

There is a list of suggestions for great snacks in Appendix A.

4.) Instead of that fast food joint, why not try a vegetarian restaurant once a week? Look for organic items.

If You Eat Well, Should You Take Vitamins?

If you are young and eat a healthy and balanced diet, you don't need to take extra vitamins and minerals. Just eating a wide variety of healthy foods will ensure an adequate supply of all the nutrients that your body needs every day.

Vitamin supplements don't offset a lousy diet. They can't neutralize excessive sugar or fat. A multi vitamin doesn't supply the wonderful disease-fighting phytochemicals in vegetables and fruits. Every year, scientists find new ingredients in food. Some fight free radicals, some clean up the circulation, some improve the immune system, some decrease the tendency for blood to clot, and still others may prevent cancer. If you don't eat a balanced diet, you miss all these constituents.

A particular vitamin is extremely important if you are deficient in that vitamin. Most of us don't scan the vitamin and mineral table to make sure that we eat foods that contain each of the twenty-eight essential nutrients every day. A typical multi-Vitamin Contains approximately twenty-three of these nutrients, skipping only those that are abundant in food and rarely lacking in the diet, such as sodium, chloride, and potassium. So, if you eat a poor diet, taking a multi vitamin is an easy way to make sure you get a sufficient amount of all of these nutrients.

If you live far from the equator, make sure that you have an adequate supply of Vitamin D during the winter months. If you do not eat meat, take supplemental Vitamin B_{12}.

Certain groups of people are known for being deficient in their intake or absorption of vitamins. Who is likely to be deficient? First, senior citizens. The elderly don't absorb nutrients from food as well as the young. Many senior citizens develop atrophic gastritis (wasting away of the stomach lining), and subsequently have trouble absorbing B_{12}. Also, they often do not consume enough calcium or Vitamin D. Second, people who don't eat properly can be deficient. These include teenagers who make poor food choices, consuming mostly soda, candy, cake, donuts, cookies, and fast food. Third, people who are on a strict diet to lose weight may also not be getting all the necessary nutrients every day. Fourth, patients suffering from anorexia nervosa or bulimia are often deficient. Fifth, patients with chronic wasting diseases that interfere with appetite, such as many cancers, cannot eat well. These groups should take a daily multivitamin with minerals.

Alternatively, these groups can take an Ensure® milkshake or Carnation Instant Breakfast® which contain an easily digestible meal along with vitamins and minerals. These are frequently recommended for patients with cancer or other diseases that interfere with proper nutrition.

Should anyone else take vitamins? Women who plan pregnancy

should take a daily pre-natal vitamin beginning four months before conception, then continue taking the vitamin through the pregnancy and for six months after the pregnancy, or as long as your obstetrician recommends. Women who receive adequate doses of folic acid are less likely to have children with neural tube birth defects than those who don't receive adequate folic acid. Also, due to the nausea and vomiting of early pregnancy, some women don't eat as well as they would like.

Women who are still menstruating should take a multivitamin that contains iron. Men and post-menopausal women usually don't need more iron than is found in the diet.

Senior adults should look for a vitamin that contains the following:

1.) 100% of the daily value of folic acid (400 mcg)

2.) 100% of Vitamin D (400 IU)

3.) At least 40% of the daily requirement of B_{12} (2.4 mcg)

Some patients have trouble swallowing the large multivitamin. One friend described his multiVitamin As a "horse pill covered with sandpaper." There's no need to choke on a vitamin pill. Unless the vitamin that you are taking is an extended release, then you can break the tablet in half and swallow the halves separately. You can also crush the tablet and mix it with a soft food such as applesauce. As a last resort, you can take a children's chewable multivitamin, although it may contain less nutrients than the adult variety.

High-priced supplements are a swindle. Buy a chain-store brand instead.

Most manufacturers change the composition of their multivitamins to keep abreast of the latest research. However, some manufacturers are slow to respond and change their formulations. A good newsletter can keep you abreast of the changes in recommendations for the content of your multivitamin.

Don't take large doses of vitamins. There are several reasons why.

First, as far as we know, your body cannot use more than the minimal daily requirement. If you are getting more than this, the rest is usually excreted in your urine.

Second, some vitamins, taken in high doses, can and do cause bodily damage. Excessive Vitamin A is capable of causing birth defects and can lead to cirrhosis and irreversible liver damage. Too much manganese can cause neurological problems. Large doses of Vitamin C can cause diarrhea. Vitamin E in large doses causes internal bleeding and hinders blood clotting in animals. These same effects are postulated in humans.

High iron levels may increase the chances of heart attack in men. Meat contains significant amounts of iron, as do beans, grains, and even some vegetables such as spinach. Many foods are fortified with iron, such as bread, cereal, and pasta. In addition, many individuals consume a daily multi vitamin with iron. These people may obtain four to five times the minimum daily requirement of that mineral. Since recent studies correlate high iron levels with heart disease, the excessive intake may be harmful.

One way to decrease the iron stores in the body is to donate blood. As a side note, donated blood is usually separated into three components, the red blood cells, the white blood cells, and the platelets, so that each donation benefits three people. Studies show that men who donate blood live longer than men who don't. Do you want to live longer and benefit humanity? Give blood.

Third, large doses of some vitamins or minerals can interfere with the absorption of other vitamins and minerals. Too much zinc can interfere with your body's absorption of copper, for example. Also, high doses of certain vitamins and minerals can interfere with the normal functioning of other vitamins and minerals in the body.

Unfortunately, some vitamin manufacturers have begun to brag about including unnecessary nutrients. Ignore these statements. Though these substances are vital to human health, they are easily supplied by a healthy diet. For example, potassium can be found in fruits and vegetables. Why would a manufacturer put a miniscule amount in the vitamin, and then list it as an ingredient? They do so in order to brag about the number of ingredients in the vitamin, as if more are better.

Unless you have a horrible diet, or have another medical problem such as severe diarrhea or vomiting, you'll get plenty of these:

Iodine	Chloride
Manganese	Biotin
Molybdenum	Boron
Sodium	Pantothenic Acid
Potassium	

The vitamin label might list some confusing substances that we don't need at all. These include the following:

Nickel

Silicon

Vanadium

Tin

When you read the vitamin label, remember that more ingredients aren't always better.

Some "nutritionists" now recommend taking a multivitamin every twelve hours. Their theory is that you will always have some antioxidants cruising around the blood stream, mopping up those rascals, the free radicals. This advice is well-intentioned but misguided. Here's why:

As noted before, the Institute of Medicine has revised the daily values previously recommended by the Food and Drug Administration. Vitamin A was revised downward from 5,000 to 3,000 IU per day. Some vitamins still contain 10,000 units. If you take a multiVitamin Every twelve hours, you will ingest 20,000 units of Vitamin A, *plus* what you receive from your food. You could easily consume five to ten times the recommended amount. Since Vitamin A has a toxicity state, taking many times the daily requirement is not a good idea.

Nature dislikes extremes. More is not better than enough. The middle way is best.

To my knowledge, no studies show any advantage to taking a multivitamin every twelve hours. Current research shows a mildly prolonged longevity for people over fifty who take a multivitamin daily.

The current belief is that antioxidants last only a few hours in the bloodstream. So, if you want to have these powerful compounds in your system most of the time, then eat fresh fruits or vegetables two to three times daily.

To summarize, taking a multivitamin once a day is a good idea if you are elderly, don't eat a balanced diet, or suffer from a disease that interferes with normal nutrient intake or absorption. Also, women who are pregnant or planning to get pregnant should take a pre-natal vitamin.

Just remember, nothing takes the place of eating a healthy diet.

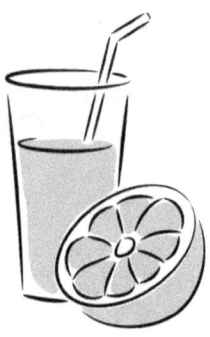

Chapter Six – Water, Juices, and Fluids

There's an incredible array of fluids available for our consumption – water, juice, herbal and caffeinated tea, alcoholic beverages, and power drinks, not to mention those delicious, expensive concoctions found at your local coffee house or the beverage shop at the mall. Does what you drink have an effect on your health, weight, energy level, or mood? The answer to all of these questions is an emphatic "yes." Let's take a look at different beverages, starting with the grandfather of them all - water.

Water

During a recent trip to Europe, I was browsing in a used book store in the city of Budapest. In a little book that called itself a "book of wisdom," I found the following quote:

"Good water, good life; bad water, bad life; no water, no life."

To this day, I haven't been able to determine the author. But I don't think I could have phrased this sentiment better myself.

When we think of nutrition, many of us think of food alone. We often overlook fluids. Next to the air we breathe, water is the most important element in our body. We breathe ten to fifteen times a minute, nine hundred times an hour, over twenty-one thousand times a day. But, did you also realize, that, depending on your age, water comprises fifty to seventy percent of all your tissues, with the highest percentages seen in babies? Your blood is fifty-five percent water and you are at least half water!

One of the most vital ingredients in any sound diet is a source of clean, healthy drinking water. If you eat well but have a lousy source of drinking water, especially one full of contaminants or pollutants, then much of your body becomes contaminated or polluted. It then performs poorly: it's like driving a beautiful car with one spark plug misfiring. No matter how well the other plugs work, that misfiring spark plug makes the car sputter and backfire. In the same way, you can breathe clean air and eat healthy food, but, if you drink bad water, you won't function optimally. This is most obvious in the impoverished countries of Africa, where inhabitants who are victims of malnutrition, war, or drought, have only terrible sources of drinking water. Even children are found drinking the water found in puddles on the ground or from rivers contaminated with multiple types of pollutants. When aid workers arrive, their first project is to dig a well to provide a source of clean water. How fortunate most of us are to live in countries where we don't even think about the safety and purity of our water before turning on the tap.

Even if we have a source of good water, how much should we drink daily? Many books and articles on nutrition have a simple dictum that reads, "Drink eight glasses of water a day." Eight is the magic number. After reading dozens of articles on water, I can't find a source for this statement. No one knows where the number eight came from. Perhaps one of the first books on nutrition came up with the number eight. Many writers since have said, "Hmmm, that sounds good," adding it to their book. But is it correct?

A short phrase in the Boy Scout manual from the 1950s read: "Water is good for you. Drink lots." The manual never presumed to tell us how much "lots" meant.

Is it necessary to drink lots of fluids? The brief answer is that it's important to drink adequate fluids, for several reasons.

Simply stated, drinking adequate fluids keeps our body in a state of proper hydration. Since fifty to sixty percent of our body is made of water, we must replenish this with a constant fresh supply. We continuously lose small amounts of fluids through our skin when we sweat and through our lungs when we breathe. These are called "insensitive losses," since we're not generally aware of them.

Drinking adequate fluid replenishes the water in our circulatory system. Remember that the blood stream delivers adequate fluid, nutrients, and oxygen to every cell in our body. When we are fully hydrated, our kidneys are most able to rid the circulation of toxins and send them to the bladder for elimination. Fluid hydrates both the blood and lymphatic circulatory systems.

Many patients who are sick, even with a sore throat, present to the physician with a variety of signs and symptoms including a rapid heart rate, called *tachycardia*. Dehydration depletes the blood of its water component, causing the blood to be concentrated and making the heart work harder and faster to deliver adequate nutrients and oxygen to the tissues. We have a saying in medicine that states, for every one degree Fahrenheit rise in body temperature, the heart rate increases ten beats per minute. We need more fluids when we are sick, a time when most of us don't feel like drinking at all.

In the old days, a professional athlete could lose ten to fifteen pounds during a hard workout on a hot day – all water weight lost through the lungs and skin, through breathing and sweating, plus the normal urine output. Nowadays, the same athlete knows to replace fluids as they're being lost and drinks sufficiently during any sports event.

Just drinking enough fluid, in addition to being vitally important to the health of every cell in our body, allows our heart to beat at a slower rate, making us more comfortable and decreasing stress on the body. This is especially important in times of increased need, such as illness or exercise,

Good hydration decreases our chances of certain ailments, including kidney stones. The very first treatment of kidney stones, regardless of the chemical composition of the stones, is to instruct the patient to drink two liters of fluid daily, diluting and washing out this small gravel while it's tiny and before it has time to solidify and grow. Someone who drinks plenty of water may also decrease the incidence of bladder cancer, since any contaminants in the urine will be more dilute and will be urinated out more often, with less time in contact with the sensitive bladder lining. Interestingly, cigarette smokers have higher incidences of bladder cancer than non-smokers.

Similarly, mucus in our nose, throat, breathing passages, and sinuses contains antibodies that help to trap bacteria and viruses. If you're dehydrated, you can't form adequate tenacious mucus.

Adequate hydration has even more benefits. Water helps with digestion and metabolism. Drinking adequate fluids prevents consti-

pation. Proper hydration keeps the skin from drying out and wrin-
kling, helping to prevent you from becoming a "prune face" before
your time.

Experts who advise drinking so much fluid often forget that not
everyone has easy access to clean water. When I was a teenager growing up in Cleveland, the Cuyahoga River was the color of rust, stunk
badly, and was so polluted that no fish could live in it. The river even
caught on fire at one time, which is ridiculous, come to think about
it - a river burning. The city became a running joke for the comedians
who made numerous jokes about the burning river. Unfortunately,
the pumping station that delivered our drinking water was located in
Lake Erie just north of where the Cuyahoga River empties into it. So,
should you drink eight glasses a day of this water? Obviously not.

Fortunately, the Cuyahoga River is much cleaner now and the
fish have come back. The water is cleaner and purer. The water in
Lake Erie is now near drinking quality *without* treatment. I drink fair
amounts of this water unfiltered every day. However, I will wager that
most readers have no idea how clean their water is or if it contains any
of the pollutants that we know to be harmful to health.

So, in a nutshell, what is the key concept regarding fluids? The key
concept is to drink adequate healthy fluids, especially water, which
should come from the purest source possible.

How can you know that your water is from a pure source?

In the United States, every municipal water department in the
country is under strict guidelines mandated by the federal government regarding the allowable amounts of many toxins. Municipal
water is tested every day for chemical contaminants and for disease-
causing microbes (like the bacteria E. Coli, found in feces, which
recently caused hundreds of people who ate contaminated spinach to
become sick in the United States). If you live in a city, the easiest way
to determine the quality of your water is to call the water department
and ask for a brochure that lists the levels of all contaminants and pollutants from the latest test results.

Many city water departments check for the following:

Metals: Copper and lead.

Inorganic Contaminants: Barium, chromium, nickel,

nitrate, thallium.

Organic contaminants: Herbicides, pesticides, and by-products of industrial processes and petroleum production.

Radioactive materials: Natural or man-made, such as byproducts of mining, gas, and oil production.

Microbial contaminants: Viruses, bacteria, and cryptosporidium

Interestingly, there are much tighter federal guidelines on public water, like your tap water, than there are on private, bottled water. Commercial water is not regulated nearly as well and is not necessarily a bargain. In fact, the International Bottled Water Association says that one fourth of all bottled water is city water. That's right, one fourth. The producers simply take city water, filter it, bottle it, and put a brand name on it. Of course, they charge a large fee for the service. My mother drank bottled water for years and died of cancer of the pancreas at the age of sixty. My father has always drunk tap water and is still alive at seventy-nine. Unless I'm in a foreign country where I don't trust the local tap water, I don't buy bottled water. Often you're simply enriching a company to perform an extremely simple maneuver.

Well water can be an excellent source of water or can be riddled with contaminants, depending on any commercial, agricultural, or industrial pollutants and solvents that leach into it. If you use well water, have it commercially tested.

Some recent articles have questioned whether the chlorine that's added to virtually all city water is harmful. From my research, I can find no reason for concern. The amount of chlorine in city water is quite small. The chlorine serves the extremely useful purpose of cleaning the water of harmful organisms. However, some authorities recommend drinking water without chlorine, preferably water bottled in hard, not soft, plastic containers, as components from the soft plastic can leach into the water.

An alternative is to use a chlorine filter with tap water. However, this may also remove beneficial additives like fluoride. Carbon filters work well to remove chlorine from water at room temperature, 50 – 80° Fahrenheit. At higher temperatures, carbon filters become ineffective and the filter itself may release contaminants into the water. So, don't use a carbon filter with hot water.

Boiling water vigorously in an open pot for five minutes removes most of the chlorine. The container must be uncovered or chlorine gas will simply collect on the lid, condense, and fall back into the water. Also, you can let tap water sit in an open container (again, uncovered). Most of the chlorine (approximately seventy-five to eighty percent), will dissipate within twenty-four hours. People with tropical fish know this technique.

For more information on water treatment, contact the NSF International (formerly the National Sanitation Foundation) at 1-877-867-3435, or online at http://www.nsf.org.

Ultimately, the choice is yours whether or not to drink water that is chlorinated.

Here are my recommendations regarding water use.

If you drink tap water, drink cold water and use cold water to prepare food or tea. Hot water may save you a few cents for the gas needed to heat the water, either in the water heater or on the stove. But the hot water from your tap has been sitting in the hot water tank for hours and may have picked up impurities there.

So, use cold water for drinking and cooking, and let the cold tap water run for a minute or so, until it feels cooler to the touch. Doing so clears the lines of any standing water that may have picked up impurities, such as lead, from old pipes. This is especially important if you live in an old building and in the morning if you haven't used water all night.

Also, some of my patients give their growing babies and children only bottled water. I recommend at least one glass of fluoridated water daily to help developing teeth to grow healthy and strong. Virtually all tap water is fluoridated. Bottled water is not. If in doubt, contact your local water department, their number can be found in the telephone book.

So, we'll assume that you've confirmed that you have a source of safe, healthy drinking water, free of impurities, insecticides, metals, and microbes. Then, you ask, just how much water is adequate? There are several ways to determine how much water you need.

First, for a specific estimate, take your weight in pounds, divide by two, and then drink that many ounces of water daily. For example, a one hundred fifty pound person would drink seventy-five ounces daily, minimum. That's about eight glasses, each holding nine ounces. Perhaps this is where the "eight glasses a day" recommendation originated.

Second, for the average size adult weighing about seventy kilograms or one hundred sixty pounds, drink the proverbial eight glasses on each day of moderate exertion. Of course, you need more if your insensitive losses – that is, the water lost through skin and lungs – are higher. Your insensitive losses will be higher if you exercise, work a physical job, have a fever, or sweat a lot.

Third, as I like to tell my patients, drink enough liquids so that your urine is the color of tap water – that is, clear. This is the easiest way to tell if you are properly hydrated. You should urinate every few hours. If your urine is deep amber or appears concentrated, you are still dehydrated. Remember that there may be a lag time of an hour or two between a sudden loss of body fluids and the urine turning darker. These sudden losses occur with intensive exercise, when bodily fluids are lost through perspiration and respiration. Gastrointestinal illnesses can cause a loss of bodily fluids through vomiting or diarrhea. Patients with a fever lose more fluids from increased sweating and from a higher respiratory rate.

Checking the color of your urine works well when you are healthy or sick. This works well when you are healthy or sick. By drinking enough fluids to keep your urine clear, you replace your lost body fluids. When you are dehydrated, one of the body's first compensatory mechanisms is to decrease fluid lost through the kidneys. When you drink adequately, you allow your kidneys to filter the blood properly.

There are people who can't rely on this method. These people can't drink fluids until their urine is clear, since they suffer from congestive heart failure, a condition in which the heart doesn't pump the blood efficiently. Drinking enough fluids to keep their urine clear may lead to an overload of water in the circulatory system and lead to a backup of fluid into the lungs, a condition termed *pulmonary edema*.

I remember visiting my grandparents shortly after I began medical school. My grandfather, who had previously sustained a heart attack, suffered from congestive heart failure. Since he was a retired farmer, he loved to quench his thirst by eating tomatoes liberally sprinkled with salt. He would sit on the porch on a hot summer night with tomatoes in one hand and a salt shaker in the other. One night, shortly after eating several tomatoes in this fashion, he became increasingly short of breath. We rushed him to the emergency room. The doctor diagnosed an overload of fluids and gave my grandfather an intravenous dose of a strong diuretic. The doctor then left my grandfather alone behind the curtain with a plastic urinal hanging over the metal rail of the gurney. After urinating briskly several times, grandpa felt well enough to go home. When they gave him his discharge instructions, he remarked that no one had ever told him to be careful with salt before.

The sodium in table salt helps to pull fluids into the bloodstream. And as we can see from the table of vegetables, tomatoes are ninety-five percent water. The combination of salt and water to a patient with congestive heart failure is like the potent one-two punch to a boxer. Down they go. We've already learned how many processed foods in the grocery store are loaded with salt.

So, a fourth way to watch your fluid status, best for those with congestive heart failure, is to know your normal weight and stick to it. I instruct patients to buy a good scale and weigh themselves in the morning. Later, if they feel short of breath or their ankles swell, they can check their weight while wearing the same amount of clothes. If they've gained more than two pounds *over* their normal weight, there is almost certainly extra water in their system. They may need an extra dose of their diuretic. Since they will pee out extra potassium with the water pill, I advise them to take an extra potassium pill along with the diuretic. Similarly, if they feel tired or dry, check their weight. If they are more than two pounds *under* their normal weight, they are probably mildly dehydrated. Drinking a glass of fluid will help.

Checking the urine color is a quick, simple way to check hydration status in healthy people without medical problems. If you suffer from congestive heart failure, buy a good scale and check your weight daily. Of course, follow this routine after consulting with your doctor. Patients with kidney problems must also consult their doctor about fluid intake.

An alternative way to get enough fluids is to eat plenty of foods that are rich in water. A glance at the tables in Appendix C will show you that these are fruits and vegetables. Not only will you restore your depleted fluids, but you'll also gain the benefit of the vitamins, minerals, and fiber in the food. You can't find a healthier way to replace your fluids than having a bowl of fresh fruit for one of your daily snacks and a salad loaded with a variety of vegetables for the other.

Juices are an alternative to fruits or vegetables. Let's look at them.

Juices

A small glass of juice (one hundred grams or three and one-half ounces) contains a modest amount of calories, from a low of seventeen for tomato juice to a high of seventy-one for prune. Juices contain virtually no fat or protein, only carbohydrates, almost all of which are sugars. Diabetics need to exercise caution here. Tomato juice is by far the lowest in sugar, which may be one reason people tend to think of the tomato as a vegetable rather than a fruit. According to botanists, the tomato is a fruit.

Fruit juices are a great source of potassium, helpful to those who need extra amounts of this electrolyte in their diet, such as patients taking a *diuretic* (the medical name for a "water pill" that increases urine output). Unless salt is added, fruit juices are extremely low in sodium. All contain modest amounts of calcium and phosphorous, plus small amounts of many other vitamins and minerals.

Some nutrients are lost in going from the fruit to the juice. Apple juice contains less fiber, Vitamin C, and folate than the fruit itself; orange juice contains less fiber, calcium, and selenium than the oranges themselves. Interestingly, the grams of water changes relatively little. Most fruits and fruit juices are eighty to ninety-five percent water. So, both the juice and the fruit are good means to replace lost body fluids.

My recommendation is that, if possible, you eat the fruit rather than just drinking the juice. That way, you'll consume all the juice plus the flesh of the fruit, so you'll get more fiber and nutrients.

Drinking juice is healthier than drinking soda pop. Rather than grabbing a can of soda for your afternoon pick-me-up, reach for a glass of juice. Most patients find that they have more energy after making the switch from soda to juice.

The best juice is made from fresh fruit, home-squeezed with a juicer. You can eat the pulp, if you wish, and you will imbibe more of the vitamins, minerals, and fiber. If you purchase the juice, look for juices that say "not from concentrate" and contain lots of pulp. If the juice is derived from concentrate, look for containers that say "100% Juice." Some "juice drinks" actually contain only fifteen to thirty percent juice. They'll tell you this at the top of the ingredient label. Look for it.

Avoid juice in metal containers as the metal may react with the acid in the juices.

If possible, buy juices with no added sugars and no artificial sweeteners.

Some juices are relatively poor in nutrients. These include grape, apple, and pear juice. Avoid them unless you're drinking for flavor. When you buy a mixed juice, check the list of ingredients. Avoid those that use these fruits as their main source of juice.

GOOD JUICES

Grapefruit

Orange

Pineapple

Prune

Cranberry

Mixed juices that say 100% juice and whose main ingredients are not grape, apple, or pear juice.

NUTRIENT-POOR JUICES

Grape

Apple

Pear

Coffee and Tea

Recent research on coffee has not borne out the earlier warnings that coffee is harmful to your health. The current recommendation is that three to four cups a day are permissible. Allow me to give you my thoughts.

I have several reservations about coffee. First, caffeine is a known stimulant. The average eight-ounce cup of coffee contains 100 milligrams of caffeine. The twelve-ounce cup of specialty coffee from some popular coffee houses can contain a walloping 300 milligrams of caffeine, an amount that would have many people flying around the ceiling. Caffeine can increase the body's production of adrenalin, causing the patient to feel "hyper," followed by a "crash," or a feeling of fatigue and low energy.

Many people become physically dependent on caffeine, a potent stimulant. When they stop drinking coffee, they experience several days of withdrawal symptoms, which include irritability, headache, and sleepiness. Second, neither the Mediterranean nor Japanese diets nor the diets of our role models include coffee. Third, coffee in high doses, more than four cups a day, has the following side effects:

1.) Heart disturbances, including rapid or irregular heart beat
2.) Increase in uric acid, which can lead to kidney stones or gout attacks
3.) Heartburn or increased acid reflux
4.) Increased excretion of the body salts, including calcium, potassium, and magnesium, substances important to maintain the body's acid-base balance and homeostasis in the blood stream.
5.) Worsening of osteoporosis.

So, patients with heart disease, high blood pressure, gout, ulcers, heartburn, or osteoporosis shouldn't drink coffee. Patients who experience the side effects of coffee, such as rapid heart rate, jitteriness, irritability, or fatigue, also shouldn't drink coffee. If you do drink coffee, have three or less cups per day. If it makes you jittery, switch to decaffeinated coffee. Alternatively, you can drink herbal tea or water.

Caution is necessary when you use any caffeinated drinks. A twelve ounce cola beverage contains forty to seventy mg. A cup of green tea has about thirty mg. Herbal tea contains no caffeine. As noted, caffeine can cause a fine tremor, rapid heart rate, and a feeling of nervousness or excitability that interferes with sleep. If you experience this, decrease your caffeine consumption. Also, drinking caffeine within three hours of sleep may interfere with a restful night.

Here are some common beverages and their caffeine content:

Beverage	Caffeine Content (Milligrams)
Water	0
Herbal tea, 8 ounces	0
Green tea, 8 ounces	30 – 40 (depending on strength)
Black tea, 8 ounces	50
Decaf coffee, 8 ounces	5-10
Regular coffee, 8 ounces	100 – 200 (depending on strength)
Cola, 12 ounces	40 - 70
Diet cola, 12 ounces	48

Green tea is a significant part of the Japanese diet. Early research indicated that green tea has several health benefits, including less cancer. Later research hasn't confirmed that green tea reduces the risk of any cancers, including breast cancer, as was earlier surmised. The final verdict simply isn't in.

However, you may feel more relaxed and less hurried when adding a warm drink to your meal. Your digestion may improve and you may feel calmer if you drink tea. Perhaps the tea will add some of the tranquility that is so highly valued in Japanese culture. Indeed, there are entire books of Zen philosophy written about the elegance of the tea ceremony. Significantly, tea adds no calories.

Alcohol

Here is a summary of the government recommendations for the consumption of alcohol:

Those who choose to drink alcoholic beverages should do so sensibly and in moderation. Drinking in moderation is considered to be up to one drink per day for women and up to two drinks per day for men. A drink is one ounce of hard liquor, four ounces to six of wine, or twelve ounces of beer.

Alcoholic beverages should not be consumed by some individuals, including:

Those who can't restrict their alcohol intake.

Women of childbearing age who may become pregnant.
Pregnant and lactating women.
Children and adolescents.
Individuals taking medications that can interact with alcohol.
Those with specific medical conditions.
Individuals engaging in activities that require attention, skill, or coordination, such as driving or operating machinery.

Those are the government recommendations. Note that alcohol interacts with many medications that can make you drowsy. These medicines include tranquilizers, sleeping pills, antihistamines, narcotics, and many others. Alcohol plus one of these medicines can create a deadly combination. Fatigue is now considered one of the leading causes of automobile accidents. The combination of alcohol, a sleepy medicine, and driving can easily equal death.

The excessive use of alcohol is also associated with traffic accidents, industrial accidents, drowning, falls, domestic violence, homicides, suicides, and date rape. The modest increase in health benefits is not worth this tremendous cost in human misery.

My recommendation is that, if you don't drink, don't start. If you do drink, limit your intake to one drink per day. Recent research indicates that the healthiest way to consume alcohol is to drink one glass of red wine with dinner.

The Fluid Pyramid

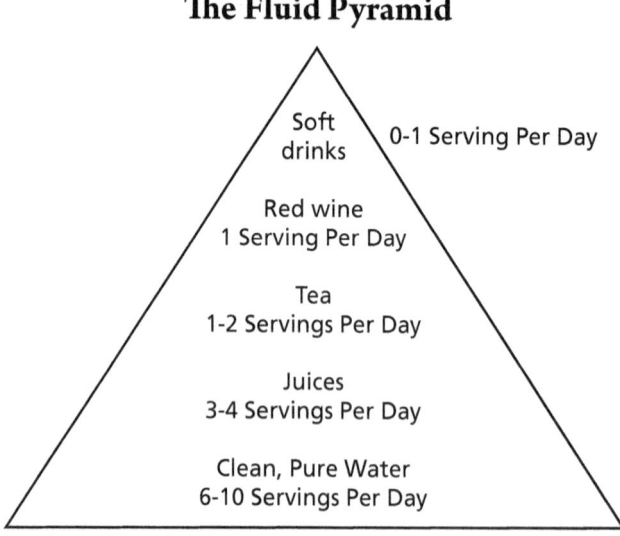

This pyramid may give you some idea of how much fluid to consume daily. This is for an average size adult with no medical problems.

Serving sizes for fluids:

Water, four to eight ounces.

Juices, four ounces.

Tea, eight ounces (one cup)

Red wine: four ounces. (If you substitute another alcoholic beverage, then use beer, twelve ounces, or hard liquor, one ounce).

Soft drinks: The less the better. One twelve-ounce can per day is more than enough.

A Great Use for Water – Brushing your Teeth

Many infectious disease experts and cardiologists now feel that the bacteria in our mouth contribute to various diseases, including bodily infections and heart disease. There is increasing evidence that proper care of the teeth can prevent heart disease. There is even new evidence that good oral hygiene may decrease the chances of some cancers. So, why not brush your teeth at least twice a day, perhaps after meals, when the bacteria count is highest? My dentist recommends using toothpaste with fluoride and tartar control.

Flossing your teeth at least once a day will remove food and bacteria between the teeth, an area hard for the toothbrush to reach. The best time to floss is before bed. If you brush and floss before retiring for the night, you will have clean teeth for eight hours.

The best routine is to floss, brush, and use a mouthwash that helps remove plaque. Your mouth will feel better, you'll stop seeding bacteria into the blood stream, and you'll live longer. The good breath certainly won't hurt your social life.

Soda is known to erode the enamel on teeth, making them more prone to cavities and more sensitive to cold. If you still drink soda pop, make sure and brush your teeth afterward. If you can't brush, at least rinse your mouth thoroughly with water. Other foods that irritate the teeth are highly acidic foods, such as orange or grapefruit juice, and foods that are high in sugar, such as candy and pastries. Many patients can eliminate their need for a sensitive toothpaste if they brush or rinse after eating or drinking any of these foods.

A Simple Way to Cut Calories

In the United States, the average person obtains about twenty percent of their daily calories from beverages. Studies show that, when you consume calories from beverages, you don't compensate by ingesting less calories later on. The latest fads in beverages are often loaded with calories. Smoothies, coffee with sugar and whipped cream, and specialty drinks contain far more calories and far less nutrition than fruit.

One way to lose weight is to confine your daily fluids to water and two eight-ounce glasses of skim milk. However, if you eat a diet that includes adequate food sources of calcium and Vitamin D, then you can save a whopping twenty percent of your daily intake of calories by confining your beverages to "free choices," those that contain no calories. These include water, coffee or tea with no sugar or cream, and diet drinks.

Since we have separate physiological mechanisms to satisfy our thirst and our hunger, drinking water doesn't tend to change your food intake later. So, you shouldn't compensate by eating more food.

In other words, what you drink doesn't tend to affect what you eat. So why not drink no calories? If you want to lose weight, why not talk with a nutritionist about an adequate diet, and then drink only water or other free beverages?

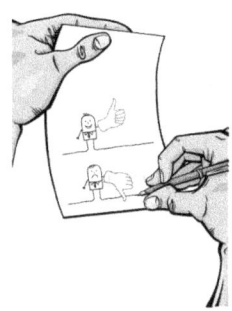

Chapter Seven – Evaluating Other Diets

Overwhelmed by Diet Books

Every year, dozens of new diet books are published. People with respectable credentials, such as doctors, nurses, researchers, nutritionists - even self-help gurus with no particular qualifications, publish a book and tout a new diet guaranteed to let you live longer, feel stronger, and be healthier than any previously published diet. They all sound great on paper. Some even claim to have the research to back them up.

How can the average person know if the new diet is any good? Should you try one of these new-fangled diets? Or are they all much ado about nothing? What's an intelligent person to do with the barrage of new books that hit the shelves every year?

Well, simply by applying the knowledge you have gleaned from this book, you can evaluate virtually any diet.

What are the qualifications of a good diet? They are four in number. The first two are from Chapter Two, where you learned to evaluate your needs. The next two are from Chapters Three through Five, where you learned to distinguish healthy from unhealthy foods. Let's take at look at our four rules:

First, a good diet must provide adequate calories for your daily energy needs, divided properly among carbohydrates, fats, and proteins, in roughly the recommended proportions, that is, 50% carbohydrate, 30% protein, and 20% fat. The amount of calories should be sufficient to maintain your ideal weight.

Second, a good diet provides all the micro nutrients, or vitamins and minerals that your body needs. As we know, the best way to ensure adequate consumption is to eat a wide variety of healthy foods. Here we must be particularly careful of those diets that eliminate an entire food group, for example, meat or fruit.

Third, a good diet doesn't include foods that are harmful to you, especially those high in saturated fat. (See the "Bad" and "Ugly" lists in this book.) As a corollary, a good diet shouldn't include food that is mostly "filler," like refined flour and soda. A good diet avoids foods that are high in sugar, salt, harmful oils, and caffeine. Alcohol should be consumed in moderation or not at all.

Fourth, a good diet includes lots of the healthy foods high in fiber, whole grains, fruits, vegetables, beans, nuts, and fish.

To summarize, a healthy diet passes four tests:

1.) Adequate calories, divided properly among carbohydrates, fats, and proteins.
2.) Adequate vitamins and minerals.
3.) Minimal bad or ugly foods.
4.) Lots of healthy foods.

Simple, huh? Let's evaluate a few common diets.

Types of Vegetarian Diets

First, let's clear up the terminology since these terms are used differently in various books.

A *vegetarian* is an individual who doesn't eat any meat, poultry, or seafood, that is, the flesh of any animal. A vegetarian can eat all plant-based oils but wouldn't eat lard or animal fat. A *lacto vegetarian* adds dairy foods to a vegetarian diet, an *ovo vegetarian* adds eggs to the vegetarian diet, and a *lacto ovo vegetarian* adds both dairy products and eggs.

A *vegan* also eliminates anything that an animal produces, such as dairy products and eggs. Remember that a vegan has completely eliminated several vital food groups. A vegan eats no meat, poultry, fish, dairy products, or eggs. As an aside, vegans are well-advised to take a daily multivitamin and to see a nutritionist to ensure adequate intake of all the necessary nutrients missing from this restricted diet.

Let's examine the nutritional components of a lacto ovo vegetarian diet.

Studies indicate that vegetarians have lower morbidity and mortality from coronary artery disease, hypertension, and several types of cancer, including lung, colon, and possibly breast cancer. But is a vegetarian diet a healthy diet?

Under our first criterion, adequate calories divided properly among carbohydrates, proteins, and fats, a sensible vegetarian diet passes the grade. A vegetarian diet will be low in saturated fat, but can contain enough fat, derived from oil, nuts, and other good fats.

Under our second criterion, the diet must provide all the necessary nutrients. Vegetarians need to be careful because they eliminate many of the foods that are rich in Vitamin B_{12}, Vitamin D, calcium, and iron. However, the first three can be obtained from milk. Iron can be obtained from a variety of non-meat foods, including beans and some vegetables, such as spinach. Let's look at each of these four nutrients.

Vitamin B_{12} is found only in animal sources. However, dairy products, including milk and ice cream, contain some B_{12}, as do eggs. Studies show that lacto ovo vegetarians have low blood levels of Vitamin B_{12}. So, a supplement is recommended in the amount of the minimum daily requirement for all vegetarians. Fortunately, since the daily requirements of B_{12} are small and it is stored and recycled by the body, deficiency of this vitamin is rare and takes years to develop.

Vitamin D is plentiful in sunny areas due to the conversion in the skin. However, vegetarians who live far from the equator will need to obtain Vitamin D from fortified dairy products such as milk. Calcium is naturally occurring and plentiful in milk. Eggs contain both calcium and Vitamin D.

The iron in plants is non-heme iron (not derived from blood). Non-heme iron isn't absorbed by the body as well as iron from animal sources. Interestingly, both vegetarians and non-vegetarians have similar rates of iron-deficiency anemia. Non-meat sources of iron include beans, especially soybeans, and certain vegetables, such as artichokes, asparagus, kale, peas, and spinach. So, vegetarians can absorb sufficient iron from their food. Notably, foods rich in Vitamin C and Vitamin C supplements increase the absorption of iron from food. Vegetarians who are iron-deficient should add a source of Vitamin C to their meals that contain some iron.

Our third criterion recommends avoiding harmful foods. This

depends on the individual vegetarian. Since a vegetarian diet is generally lower in calories, a vegetarian must consume enough other foods to make up for the calories that are not available from calorie-dense foods such as fatty meats. If the vegetarian consumes high levels of unhealthy foods such as bleached white flour, sugar, salt, and hydrogenated oils, say, in the form of cakes, cookies, donuts, soda pop, candy, and other snacks, then much of the nutritional benefit of being a vegetarian may be lost. Some teenage patients proudly proclaim their vegetarian status. However, on further questioning, one finds that many of the foods that they consume are junk foods. This is not a healthy change.

On the other hand, if a sensible vegetarian eats lots of fruits, vegetables, whole grains, beans, peas, and nuts, then the diet can be very healthy indeed. Our fourth criterion has been met. However, even the lacto ovo vegetarian loses the benefits of consuming fish. Ongoing research continues to indicate that fish are a valuable component of a healthy diet.

The Ornish Diet

The Ornish diet is vegetarian. The dieter consumes no meat, poultry, or fish. Interestingly, the diet also excludes the consumption of oils. The diet allows the consumption of non-fat dairy products such as skim milk and egg whites but not the yolks. In essence, it's a lacto ovo vegetarian diet which excludes all milk-*fat*, egg *yolks*, and vegetable *oils*. We discussed this diet previously in the Chapter Five, "Individual Food Groups."

As with all research, the effects of the diet alone are hard to tease out for the simple fact that Ornish also has his patients simultaneously start a program of meditation and exercise. As we've seen, exercise is an important part of any healthy program and can provide collateral blood supply in the heart, opening up the smaller blood vessels that aren't usually the main channels for blood flow. Controversy exists as to whether exercise alone can reverse hardening of the arteries. Exercise does help to develop collateral circulation.

We continue to discover the marvelous abilities of meditation to heal the body. Studies at Harvard Medical School, conducted by Dr.

Herbert Benson and others, show that various forms of meditation, such as the Transcendental Meditation popular in India and Tibet, evoke powerful healthy responses in people who practice them. These responses include:

> Lower blood levels of stress hormones.
> Lower blood pressure.
> Lower heart rate and respiratory rate.
> Lower metabolic rate as measured by oxygen consumption.
> Lower lactic acid levels in the body.

These simple meditation techniques are powerful means of deeply relaxing the body, even more than sleep, while maintaining a level of alertness greater than the normal waking state. Meditation is an integral ingredient in this program and is probably responsible for some of its beneficial effects. For those patients in whom stress is a problem, the book *The Relaxation Response*, by Herbert Benson, is highly recommended.

Aside from the benefits of exercise and meditation, how does this diet stack up against our four criteria?

Criterion one, are adequate calories properly divided among carbohydrates, proteins, and fats? The fat content, especially saturated fat, is extremely low, with more calories coming from carbohydrates. However, the patients seem to have had no ill effects from this proportion.

Criterion two requires the presence of all micro nutrients. This diet fares better than a vegan diet, since non-fat dairy products are allowed. This diet provides a sufficient amount of calcium. Iron can be obtained from non-meat sources such as whole grains, beans, spinach, beets, and other vegetable sources. Milk and dairy foods are a good source of Vitamin B$_{12}$. The diet bans all oils, which are high in natural Vitamin E, but these can be consumed in whole grains or nuts. Thus, all micro nutrient groups are represented.

Criteria three requires avoiding harmful foods. The diet bans all the fatty meats which head the list of "ugly foods." Also, dairy products high in fat, such as whole milk, cheese, and ice cream, aren't allowed. Essentially, harmful foods are absent from this diet.

Criteria four involves eating a wide variety of healthy foods. The diet promotes lots of fruits, vegetables, and whole grains, all very healthy. No fish are allowed, which is a possible problem, but the benefit of omega-3 fatty acids can be obtained from walnuts, flax seeds, and other vegetable sources noted previously. Some researchers feel that the consumption of fish confers specific health benefits not found in any plant-based foods, but further study is needed.

On the whole, this diet fares well under our criteria, especially since low-fat dairy products are allowed, which avoids the possible problems of low calcium and B_{12} consumption seen with a strict vegan diet. My own opinion is that most people fare better adding some healthy fish to the diet. Extremely active individuals such as Triathlon participants have noted more energy after adding meat back into their diet. Remember that the Ornish program includes exercise and meditation in addition to healthy eating. All three of these lifestyle changes undoubtedly contribute to the heartening results of the research. Of course, patients are instructed not to smoke.

This diet receives a good grade, particularly for people with coronary artery disease. As with any restrictive diet, some patients complain about the lack of their favorite food, particularly those who love meat or fish.

The Atkins Diet

Dr. Robert Atkins has founded a small empire with his diet books touting the revolution named after him. His diet targets carbohydrates as the source of much of the obesity in this country. In his two week induction diet, he advises his readers to order a juicy cheeseburger, throw away the bun, and eat the meat and cheese. Free foods, that is, those allowed in unlimited amounts, include all meats, all fish, all fowl, and eggs. Cream is allowed but not skim milk, sour cream but not yogurt. Dieters are allowed no fruit, bread, grains, or starchy vegetables. They are advised to be wary of sugar, corn syrup, white flour, corn starch, and many refined sugars such as maltose, dextrose, and fructose.

The diet is big on supplements, which are called vita-nutrients. These include vitamins, minerals, essential fatty acids, intermediary metabolites, and herbs.

How does this diet stack up against our criteria?

Criterion one, are adequate calories divided properly among carbohydrates, proteins, and fats? The Atkins diet is low in carbohydrate. He properly criticizes some of the carbohydrates, such as bleached white flour and the refined sugars, which aren't healthy. However, this diet is quite high in fats, especially if you indulge liberally in fatty meats. Unfortunately, the diet derives far more than twenty percent of its calories from fat and far less than fifty percent of its calories from carbohydrate.

Criterion two refers to whether the diet provides all the necessary micro nutrients. The glaring deficiency in the induction diet is the lack of fruit. We need to exercise caution with any diet that completely excludes one food group. As we have seen, fruits are high in many nutrients. They are a great source of carotenoids, folic acid, Vitamin C, potassium, and fiber. They also are water-rich, providing a nice, vitamin-healthy way to obtain fluids. However, since the diet includes supplements and liberal amounts of vegetables, most of these essential nutrients are found in sufficient amounts. My preference is that patients obtain most of their vitamins and minerals from food. As their name states, supplements are meant to "supplement," not replace, nutrients found naturally in foods.

Under criterion three, avoiding harmful foods, the diet unfortunately can't receive a good grade. The liberal use of many of the "ugly" foods, including fatty meats such as bacon, sausage, pepperoni, and other meats cured with nitrites, is unhealthy. High fat diets have been implicated in atherosclerosis and several forms of cancer.

Criterion four requires eating lots of healthy foods. The Atkins diet restricts some of the healthy, natural, nutritious food groups, such as fruits and whole grains. Many nutritionists recommend their favorite "miracle foods" which they feel carry tremendous health benefits. Most of these foods are fruits and vegetables, some are grains, none are meats. On the Atkins diet, you won't eat many of these miracle foods. Basically, only vegetables are allowed, not whole grains or fruits.

The diet also restricts low-fat dairy products. Although dairy products are somewhat controversial, many nutritionists recommend low-fat dairy products, such as skim or one percent milk and low-fat yogurt.

Furthermore, since the very low-fat Ornish diet has been shown in research studies to actually reverse hardening of the arteries, what does a high-fat diet do to the blood vessels? Wouldn't a high-fat diet promote more hardening of the arteries? Can we justify a high-fat diet? Both the Mediterranean and Japanese diets are low in saturated fat. Both of our role models, Jack La Lanne or Strom Thurmond, eat a diet high in healthy carbohydrates and low in saturated fat. The overwhelming body of evidence indicates that a healthy diet is largely plant based. Instead, the Atkins diet emphasizes lots of meat.

One current theory is that patients lose weight because they restrict carbohydrates, causing them to break down body stores of fat. This type of metabolism is called *ketosis*. Unfortunately, ketosis can cause dehydration meaning that some of the weight loss is due to the unhealthy loss of body water.

Over time, patients find out two things on the Atkins diet. First, the diet tends to become a bit monotonous. Even meat lovers get sick of a big juicy burger with no bread. Second, after about six months, weight loss hits a plateau and patients tend not to lose any more. Patients on a healthy diet (low in saturated fat and calories) tend to catch up and surpass the amount of weight lost on the Atkins diet.

Patients with diabetes should *not* be on a high protein diet such as the Atkins. Protein breaks down into waste products that must be excreted through the kidneys - just what diabetics don't need.

In its defense, the diet does emphasize vegetables and rightly criticizes the bleached flour and refined sugars so prevalent in American food. Dr. Atkins also recommends fish or fish oil supplements with their heart-healthy omega-3 fatty acids. Some patients unable to lose weight on other diets are successful on the Atkins diet.

These good points do not offset the other harmful aspects of the diet. Being able to lose weight does NOT mean that your diet is healthy. You can be a bean pole and still have severe hardening of the arteries. The story of John the maintenance man in the beginning of this book is an excellent case in point. This diet does not lower your susceptibility to the two biggest killers, heart attack and stroke.

Patients frequently ask to start this diet for two reasons. One, they get to eat the meat that they love. Second, they tend to lose weight during the first couple of months. Their feeling is that they can "jump start" their weight loss, then switch to a healthier diet. My feeling is that there are healthier ways to lose weight. I agree to follow their progress clinically, with the understanding that they will discontinue this diet promptly after one to two months.

The Zone Diet

Dr. Barry Sears has soared to popularity with his Zone Diet. He has written eight books at the latest count, each giving a different twist on this particular diet. His initial books were quite complex, using difficult formulas to explain how to balance your intake. His later books have simplified the results of his research to make it easier to understand, remember, and apply.

Dr. Sears recommends balancing your diet among the three macro nutrient groups (carbohydrates, proteins, and fats) at each meal. He differentiates between good and bad types of food in each of the three groups. This is a sound idea since there are good and bad carbohydrates, good and bad fats, and good and bad proteins. He properly touts the value of nuts as a healthy choice for fats.

In a later book, he recommends his Top 100 Foods, making it easier to find the healthy choices in each of the three food groups. He has simplified food selection with his easy rule for filling your plate. His advice is to cover two-thirds of the plate with healthy carbohydrate, one-third with healthy protein, and sprinkle healthy fat over the top. This suggestion is not too far from our own rule on how to cover your plate.

However, Sears may have prematurely taken the glycemic index of foods at face value, forgetting that much important research on this field continues to this day. Also, he excludes some foods that are clearly beneficial. For example, among his Top 100 Foods, the only whole grains that make the grade are barley and oats. There is no mention of whole grain brown rice, whole grain corn, or even whole grain wheat. He doesn't list some clearly healthy vegetables, such as carrots, perhaps because of his tendency to judge foods based on their glycemic index. Only olive oil makes his Top 100 Food list, to the exclusion of canola, soybean, and oils derived from nuts. He says little about the body's ability to digest the components of cow's milk. Also, there seems to be a new Zone diet book every year, way past the point of saturation.

Regarding our four criteria:

Criterion one, balance of calories: The Zone Diet excels with its adequate calories properly divided among carbohydrates, proteins, and fats.

Criterion two, providing all micro nutrients: Since there are no severe restrictions, as in a vegan diet, the Zone diet provides an ample supply of all micro nutrients.

Criterion three, avoiding harmful foods: The Zone diet includes none of the "ugly foods" mentioned in our list of 'The Good, The Bad, And the Ugly." Dr. Sears wisely avoids the use of fatty meats, bleached white flour, and virtually all of the junk food that so many people eat to excess.

Criterion four, eating lots of healthy foods: The diet passes this test also, since the Top 100 recommended foods are healthy.

On the whole, this is a well-researched and nutritious diet.

Now that you have these four criteria in hand, you can feel confident of evaluating any diet in minutes. When the latest book on nutrition hits the stands, you are empowered to apply the four criteria and see if the diet stands up. You will no longer let hucksters fool you with their impersonation of experts. Take a look at the content of the diet, apply these four criteria, and decide if it makes the grade.

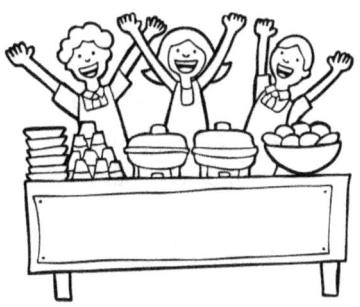

Chapter Eight -
Buying, Storing, and Preparing Food

General Principles

Buying food wisely is one of the most important activities you can undertake to ensure a nutritious, healthy diet. Ideally, you hope to find whole, natural foods, free of artificial flavors, colors, sweeteners, preservatives, and synthetic additives.

Unadulterated, unprocessed food is best. If you have the choice, pick food that isn't treated with artificial fertilizers, chemicals, or insecticides. In other words, buy organic food when it's available and affordable. Avoid artificial sweeteners, several of which have been associated with cancer in laboratory animals. When it comes to food, the closer it is to natural, the better it is for you.

Immediately after buying any food that loses potency over time (virtually all fresh food), remember the "Two C's." Keep food <u>cold</u> and <u>covered</u>. Fruits and vegetables should be eaten shortly after ripening or placed in the refrigerator. Fresh food loses its vitamin and mineral content in a matter of days. Canned food can sit on the shelf at a constant, preferably cool, temperature for months but will lose nutrient value eventually.

Wash your hands thoroughly with soap and hot water for thirty seconds before preparing food. This precaution can't be emphasized enough, especially if you're cooking for other people. Antibacterial soaps tend to dry the skin and aren't recommended. The Center for Disease Prevention and Control (CDC) recommends alcohol wash, rather than antibacterial soap, to kill bacteria on the skin. Even then, you only need to kill bacteria on your hands if you are preparing food for someone with an immune system weakened by disease, such as cancer or AIDS. If you use an alcohol wash, first wash your hands, then use an alcohol wash with at least sixty-two percent ethyl alcohol. This is the lowest concentration found to be effective at killing bacteria.

Separate raw foods from cooked or ready to eat foods. Wash your hands after working with raw foods and before working with other foods. Wash fruits and vegetables. Wash any surfaces that come in contact with the food, such as cutting boards and counter tops. Wash the cutting board in the dishwasher or with hot, soapy water. Choose cloths over sponges for your cleaning. Cloths are easier to rinse and clean. They can be washed in the laundry and air-dried on a clothes line.

Eggs

If possible, buy eggs laid by free-running hens that eat grain rather than chemically treated feed. U.S. Grade AA is best. If you know a farmer, buy eggs within one to two days of their laying. If not, buy eggs at the market, choosing a carton with the latest expiration date. Avoid raw or partially cooked eggs and foods that contain them.

Cook foods to a safe temperature for a long enough time to kill any microorganisms.

When you arrive home, store the eggs immediately in the refrigerator in a closed egg container. The egg shell is somewhat porous and can lose nutrients. The lower temperature reduces the growth of bacteria such as salmonella. Don't wash eggs before storage. Try to use the eggs within one week of purchase. Brown eggs are equal in nutritional value to white.

Milk and Yogurt

Look for skim milk or, my favorite, one percent. By skimming off the cream, we avoid the high fat content of milk. However, the natural fat-soluble vitamins are in the fat. I drink one percent milk, since I prefer getting some of the natural vitamins in the milk fat. Patients who are watching their weight, or who have a history of coronary artery disease, may wish to choose skim milk.

Refrigerate milk immediately. Every minute it sits on the kitchen table shortens its life. As with all fresh food, try to purchase milk as soon as possible after milking. Use the milk promptly, preferably within five days of purchase. Light tends to destroy the vitamins in milk. Avoid all raw or unpasteurized milk and milk products.

Plain, unflavored, low-fat yogurt is a good variety. Light yogurt contains even less calories and fat than low-fat but often includes an artificial sweetener, which isn't recommended. My advice is to avoid all artificial sweeteners. The manufacturer may add a small amount of fruit. Why not enrich the yogurt yourself by adding fresh fruit, wheat germ, or nuts? If the yogurt isn't sweet enough, add a dollop of honey or molasses. Some nutritionists suggest blackstrap molasses, which is rich in nutrients including iron and calcium. During cooking, you can substitute yogurt for cream in most recipes.

Meat

Most livestock in the United States is fed chemically treated feed rather than grain. Cattle are also given hormones, steroids, antibiotics, and occasionally tranquilizers. Meat is often preserved with nitrites and nitrates. Many meat products, such as cold cuts at the deli, still contain water, fillers, artificial flavors, spices, and, of course, preservatives.

The probability of contracting Bovine Spongiform Encephalopathy (BSE), or Mad Cow Disease, from eating beef is extremely low.

Try to buy the freshest meat available. Rather than purchase frozen meat, buy refrigerated meat and freeze it yourself. Store your raw meat and poultry on the lowest shelf of the refrigerator. This prevents leaking juices from falling onto other foods.

Never eat raw or undercooked meat or poultry. Make sure the meat is fully cooked, usually for one hour at 350° Fahrenheit. The only accurate way to determine that meat is properly cooked is with a thermometer. Although many chefs use a knife to check for sufficient cooking, this is not dependable.

Fish

Fish that you buy at a grocery store or market can be a risk since it spoils quickly. Use a reliable merchant. Purchase fish that was caught as recently as possible. Talk to the fishmonger. The fish should be springy and firm, without a spoiled odor. The flesh shouldn't be starting to separate.

Your nose may be your best guide. If the fish smells tainted, throw it out. As with meat, store fish on the lowest shelf of the refrigerator to prevent leaking juices from falling onto other foods.

Fish should be eaten within one to two days of purchase, preferably immediately. Remove the skin and the fat underneath with a sharp knife, which reduces contaminants in the fish. Bake, broil, or grill your fish on a rack. This allows the fat, in which many chemicals concentrate, to drain off. Don't sauté or fry the fish, as the fat cannot drain off. Breading and batter also trap the fat drippings.

Grains, Flour, Bread, and Pasta

Buy whole grains. White rice and refined wheat flour have been stripped of the bran and the germ, which contains Vitamin E, calcium, phosphorous, iron, B vitamins (such as thiamin and niacin), and much of the protein. Look for a variety of whole grain rice, such as brown rice, and whole or cracked wheat. Avoid bread if its ingredients include "flour," "white flour," "bleached flour," or even "wheat flour." Remember, even "unbleached flour" has been stripped of the bran and the germ. It just hasn't been bleached, or colored white. Bleached flour serves no purpose. Why would anyone need to change the nice, natural color of flour, anyway? Bleach your shirts, not your bread.

Bran, the husk of the grain, is very high in fiber. You find higher concentrations of bran in cereals than in bread or muffins.

Avoid emulsifiers, such as monoglycerides and diglycerides, which are used to soften bread. Also avoid preservatives, such as sodium and calcium propionate, which aren't necessary to preserve good quality bread. Buy your bread fresh and store it in the refrigerator. Many types of bread contain refined sugars, such as fructose, dextrose, and corn syrup. Avoid them if possible. Generally, you should recognize all the ingredients in the bread. They have names like wheat, oats, and corn.

Better yet, why not try your hand at making your own bread from whole grains? Then you can be certain that the ingredients are healthy. Sweeten them with molasses or honey if you prefer.

Pasta made from white flour is a high starch, low protein grain that has been stripped of much of its natural vitamins and fiber. After stripping the grain, the manufacturer adds synthetic vitamins and calls the product "enriched," even though it contains less nutrients than the whole grain. Pasta includes macaroni, spaghetti, lasagna, and other similar products. If the manufacturer adds egg products, the product is called a noodle. So, a noodle is pasta with egg added. In noodles, look for fresh whole eggs rather than dried eggs or egg yolks.

Corn meal should be whole and unbolted. Corn starch has lost much of its nutrient content since the germ has been removed. It's useful as a thickener but has little nutritional value.

Buying Vegetables

Fresh vegetables are your best choice. Unfortunately, the "fresh" vegetables you buy in the grocery store may already have a shelf life of two weeks or more. Each day they lose essential nutrients. Ask the grocer when the produce was picked.

Don't buy vegetables that have broken skin, bruises, punctures, or brown spots. The vegetables should look fresh and feel firm to the touch. Remember, the more colorful the vegetable, the higher the Vitamin Content.

Frozen vegetables are usually prepared quickly after harvest and make an excellent choice, as they retain much of their vitamin and mineral content. Although many companies now use the quick freezing methods described earlier, it's still difficult to tell how long the vegetables have been sitting in warehouses, trucks, or freezers. The vegetables may have been thawed and refrozen repeatedly, each time depleting more vitamins. Vegetables that are cut before packaging also lose vitamins, so choose the whole variety instead of the cut variety when possible.

Canned vegetables, if they are processed promptly after picking, also retain most of their vitamins and minerals. However, many of the same problems exist as with frozen vegetables. Canned vegetables sometimes sit for months on shelves. Few manufacturers print a legible date of manufacture on the packaging. Also, vegetables lose some Vitamin Content to water. Still, if you have a choice between canned vegetables and no vegetables, eat the canned vegetables. Choose unsalted canned vegetables. Drink the water that they come in or use it for your tea. Avoid vegetables with artificial colors.

Truly fresh produce, eaten within a few hours after picking, is the healthiest and tastiest. The best place to buy vegetables is from a roadside stand. Buy vegetables in season, immediately after harvesting. Try stopping by a roadside stand run by the farmer. Ask the family when the vegetables were picked. "Today" is the best answer.

So, the best vegetables for retaining their potency are:

> Fresh (the more recently picked, the better)
> Frozen
> Canned

The wonderful Japanese and Greek diets mentioned earlier use food prepared in this manner. Perhaps this is one reason why these people are so healthy. In fact, much of the world still consumes food promptly, with each day's meals bought that morning at the local market. Much of Europe, with a standard of living comparable to that in America, eats this way. As one nutritionist said in a seminar, she likes the way French people eat. They use fresh ingredients, purchased that day, lovingly prepared, and then shared with friends. Why not try this? Certainly, you're busy, but can you think of a better way to spend your time or to show love to your family?

Cooking Vegetables

Prolonged cooking destroys nutrients. Remember not to overcook. Vegetables lose vitamin content during boiling or sitting on the steaming trays so common in cafeterias. When heated too long, vegetables lose their crunchy texture. Fresh vegetables are crunchy; overcooked vegetables are soft.

The best way to cook vegetables is:

1.) Don't. Eat vegetables raw, as nature intended. This preserves most nutrients. Wash vegetables just before eating. Avoid raw sprouts.

2.) Microwave. Some vegetables aren't edible when raw. Microwave them long enough to be warm or edible, but no longer than necessary. Corn and asparagus, for example, cook extremely well in the microwave.

3.) Baking. This is especially good for vegetables with a skin, such as onions, potatoes, squash, and so on. Undercook rather than overcook.

4.) Steaming. Place the vegetables on a steamer over a small amount of water, boil gently, not for too long, and eat while still crunchy and fresh.

5.) Stir fry. Chinese vegetables immediately come to mind. Celery, green beans, onions, mushrooms, and broccoli, all taste great by this method. Don't overcook. Use healthy oil.

Some nutritionists feel that vegetables such as carrots may be better digested if cooked. Recent research shows that other foods, such as garlic, onions, and tomatoes, may release more of their beneficial properties if heated. You may wish to follow the research. These foods are healthy either way, so include lots of them in your diet.

Fruits

Buy fresh fruits in season, preferably from a roadside stand, where you can talk to the farmer and determine how fresh the product really is. Also, see if he sprays the fruit with pesticides. Try to find organic fruit. If you can't, choose fruit that is in its own thick skin, like watermelon, cantaloupe, honeydew, grapefruit, oranges, nectarines, lemons, limes, papaya, mango, kiwi, and pineapples. (Granted, unless you live in Florida, California, New Zealand, or South America, you won't be able to find many of these fruits at a local roadside market, since they come from warmer climates).

Imported fruits and some domestic fruits, such as cherries, grapes, strawberries, and apples, tend to be heavily sprayed. Wash them in water with a small amount of liquid dish detergent and rinse them thoroughly immediately before eating. Don't wash fruits, especially berries, until you are ready to eat them, since they decay more promptly after washing.

Some fruits, like bananas, are picked green, gassed in the warehouse to induce ripening, and then shipped to distant parts. Other fruits, such as apples, are waxed heavily to improve appearance. This artificial coloring is visible in the white part of the apple just under the skin. The leathery spots seen on the skin of some fresh apples at the local market aren't harmful.

Look for fresh fruits free of bruises, punctures, and brown spots. Give preference to those that still have the stem in the top of the fruit (like apples). Let the fruit ripen in indirect light. Direct sunlight can cause excessive ripening and depletes vitamins. Eat the fruit promptly or store it in the refrigerator when ripe.

You can find frozen fruits with no added sugar, color, flavor, or preservatives. Check the label. As usual, the fewer ingredients, the better. The best product contains only the fruit itself. Frozen fruits can be good alternatives to fresh. Canned fruits tend to lose some nutrients to the liquid.

Avoid juice and cider that is not pasteurized. These products may contain the bacteria E Coli. Every couple of years, there's an outbreak of food-borne illness usually caused by the colon bacteria of livestock that graze near farms or orchards.

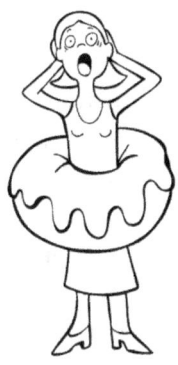

Chapter Nine – Supplements and Snacks

Supplements

Supplements are all the rage now. Many "experts" claim that their favorite supplement can increase longevity, prevent cancer, eliminate heart disease, or, perhaps most commonly, boost energy. Who among us couldn't use more energy? Americans pop over $3 billion worth of these little boosters annually. Many contain nothing more than the latest fad ingredient and a few fillers. There is no solid research to back the outrageous claims made by the promoters.

As noted before, this book recommends few supplements – a multivitamin for certain people, Vitamin D if you're unable to obtain adequate amounts from sunshine or food, and possibly fish oil capsules if you are unable to eat the whole fish. There's no solid evidence for the benefit of any other supplement. Save your hard-earned money. Let the hucksters find a real job.

No manufacturer can outdo Mother Nature. If you want to take a supplement, try one of the following. You can make your own nutritious "natural supplements" at home.

1.) Power milk shake – This is one of my favorites. Put plain low-fat yogurt (you can substitute skim or one percent milk or juice) and fresh fruit in a blender. You'll find a nice variety of fresh fruits in season and frozen fruits out of season. If you have a sweet tooth, add a little honey or molasses. If you are not allergic to them, add a handful of a variety of nuts, as they're high in nutrients and healthy fat. Within a few seconds you have a great shake.

Want even more nutrients? You can now purchase

bags containing a mixture of ten whole grains in powder form at the grocery store. Sprinkle a tablespoon or two of this powder into your milkshake. What supplement can be better than this, nature's own design?

The contents of the power milk shake are:

> Plain low fat yogurt, 4 – 8 ounces.
> Variety of fresh or frozen fruits, ½ - 1 cup.
> Variety of nuts, preferably including almonds and walnuts, ¼ - ½ cup.
> Mix containing several whole grain flours, ¼ cup.
> Place in a blender and puree to preferred consistency.

2.) Wheat germ – Loaded with B vitamins and protein, you can find wheat germ in the cereal department of the grocery store. Look for the untoasted variety since it preserves more of the vitamins. Once you open the package, store it in the refrigerator. Sprinkle the wheat germ over cereal or add a teaspoon to your power milkshake.

3.) Fruits – Have a basket of fresh fruit sitting on the table. Children and adults can munch on this rather than grab a cola drink or candy bar. For snacks, prepare a fresh fruit salad.

4.) Salad – Prepare a salad with your favorite greens, and then cover it with several different fresh vegetables. Want a great supplement? Add some low fat cheese, pine nuts, and garbanzo beans. Walnuts are good source of omega-3 fatty acids. If you need salad dressing, use vinegar and cold-pressed extra virgin olive oil or a light salad dressing. Alternatively, try a fresh or frozen vegetable medley.

5.) Nuts – Try a half cup of a variety of your favorite nuts, including almonds and walnuts. Eat them as a snack or add them to meals. You can also throw them in your milk shake.

6.) Juice – Grab a few fruits or vegetables from your refrigerator, put them in your juicer, and make a great beverage.

7.) Home made whole grain bread – Prepare your own bread at home or buy the most natural loaf you can find (try a small bakery or health food store). Eat this on its own or with fresh fruit, yogurt, or low-fat cheese. If you have trouble keeping on weight, add a slice of avocado, another food source rich in healthy fat. Those with a sweet tooth can add a small amount of honey for extra energy.

Snacks

Here are some additional ideas for a mid-morning or mid-afternoon snack:

1.) Pumpkin or sunflower seeds, unsalted.

2.) Low-fat yogurt or cottage cheese.

3.) Whole grain cereal. Many cereals are quite healthy and can be eaten as a snack. Granola tends to be high in fat.

4.) Toast with a small amount of honey.

5.) Whole grain chips with garden salsa containing tomatoes, corn, and beans.

6.) Whole grain pretzels.

7.) Yellow popcorn, cooked in a hot air popper, or low-fat microwave popcorn with no trans fat in the ingredients.

Why not power up your body with a supplement after your daily exercise. Or why not munch your snack while sitting in the sunshine for twenty minutes?

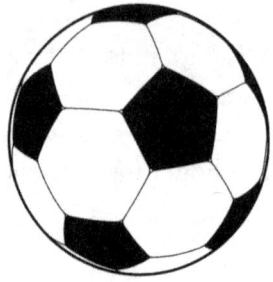

Chapter Ten – Take Good Care of Yourself

Introduction

If you've read and implemented the principles in this book, then you're already accomplishing the following:

1.) Staying within five percent of your ideal weight.
2.) Eating regular meals.
3.) Eating breakfast every day.
4.) Not smoking.
5.) Getting regular exercise.
6.) Consuming no more than one alcoholic beverage daily.
7.) Getting seven to eight hours of sleep a night.

Regarding nutrition specifically, you:

1.) Choose healthy food, meal after meal.
2.) Eat food packed with nutrients and high in fiber, consisting mostly of natural foods, especially fruits, vegetables, whole grains, nuts, beans, fish, and low-fat dairy products.
3.) Eat food that's low in calories, saturated fat, cholesterol, sugar, sodium, refined flour, artificial colors, flavors, and preservatives.
4.) Eat red meat no more than three times a week and eat no ugly meats.
5.) Drink adequate fluids to hydrate yourself, mostly water, tea, or juices.

If you've accomplished these goals, you have ninety-five percent of the picture. Congratulations.

Join the Healthiest Group

Heart disease has been the number one killer in America for years. Extensive research since the 1950s, including the long-running Framingham study, has shown that the three major risk factors for heart disease are high cholesterol, high blood pressure, and smoking. In medicine, we continue to refine our knowledge using information gleaned from these long-term studies.

Let's look at our goals for each of these three vital parameters:

Twenty years ago, a cholesterol level under 300 was considered normal. Ten years ago, a cholesterol level under 240 was considered normal. Five years ago, under 200 was good. Now we know that a cholesterol level under 150 is healthiest. Recent research has shown that people are healthiest if the LDL, the unhealthy cholesterol, is kept under 100 in most patients and under 70 in diabetic patients.

In early 2003, we felt that any blood pressure under 140 over 90 was fine. (The top number - systolic blood pressure - measures the pressure of the blood on the artery walls in millimeters of mercury when the heart is beating. The bottom number - diastolic blood pressure - measures the pressure of the blood on artery walls between heartbeats, or when the heart is relaxed). Now we know that truly healthy people have a blood pressure less than 120 over 80. Our goal now is a blood pressure reading of 115/75 in everyone.

People in the lowest risk group don't smoke.

So, here are your recommendations. Keep your total cholesterol less than 150, maintain a blood pressure less than 120 over 80, and don't smoke. So, see your doctor to have your blood pressure and cholesterol checked. If the results are higher than desired, discuss changes in diet and lifestyle with your physician, put them into practice, and monitor your progress until you reach normal levels. Make sure that you work together to reach these levels. Then you will join the people who have a mortality rate from coronary heart disease that is ninety percent lower than people who don't follow these guidelines.

There are medications for cholesterol, diabetes, and high blood pressure. In diabetics, for example, medications called statins can significantly reduce overall cardiovascular morbidity and mortality (disease and death, respectively). Half of an adult aspirin daily (or two baby aspirins) may reduce the risk of heart attack. Blood pressure medicines like ACE inhibitors significantly reduce damage to the blood vessels and help to preserve kidney function. All these medications have been available for years. Use them if your lifestyle changes don't bring about the desired levels of cholesterol and blood pressure that we discussed.

My feeling is that the natural methods of prevention described in this book are safer than medication. If there is a natural alternative, perhaps one that involves a change of lifestyle, why not give it a try? Don't choose a pill just because it is easier.

Many medications are expensive. They all have side effects, including the "safe" medicines that you can obtain over the counter. Aspirin causes intestinal bleeding. Acetaminophen can cause liver damage. No medicine is without side effects.

Serious problems, like high cholesterol and high blood pressure, present *greater* risks to your health than the side effects from the pills that treat them. Follow your doctor's advice regarding medication. If changes in lifestyle don't bring about sufficient changes in your health to put you in the healthiest group, take the medicine.

The healthiest group has the following characteristics:

Weight	Within five percent of ideal
Total cholesterol	200 mg or lower (150 is the goal)
LDL cholesterol	100 mg or lower (70 or lower if you are diabetic)
HDL cholesterol	40 mg or higher
Triglycerides	150 mg or lower
Fasting glucose	110 mg or lower
Blood pressure	120/80 in millimeters of mercury (115/75 is ideal)
Smoking	Non-smoker

See your doctor regularly. Aim for the above values using lifestyle alone if possible, medicine if necessary.

Specific Medical Problems

An incredible number of patients suffer from diabetes, obesity, and hypertension. In addition to the above, the following information may be helpful:

Diabetic Patients

Remember that the first three treatments for diabetes are diet, diet, and diet. Follow your diabetic diet carefully. There are wonderful publications available from your local hospital, nutritionist, or the American Diabetic Association to help you. Many nurses specialize in teaching diabetics. They offer helpful information and great encouragement to patients who wish to treat their diabetes naturally. See them. Educate yourself.

Don't smoke. Diabetes and smoking both damage the blood vessels, the highways of the body. Your heart pumps blood through this amazing, intricate network, delivering calories, vitamins, fluids, glucose, and energy, twenty-four hours a day, every day of your life. No damage is more insidious than slowly destroying your blood vessels. Diabetes is still the number two cause of blindness and kidney failure in patients from advanced nations. One of the rarest patients in medicine is an elderly diabetic smoker, for the simple reason that they die young. So, if you meet one, offer congratulations. They've won the lottery. Any diabetic who smokes is playing Russian roulette.

Keep your blood vessels open by getting regular exercise. At the very least, take a brisk walk for half an hour daily.

Eat whole grains rather than processed flour.

Eat smaller portions.

Decide how much you will cheat.

Know the nutritional values of different foods. Eat more fruits that are low in sugars and high in fiber (rhubarb, raspberries, blackberries).

Eat more vegetables than fruits. Choose those lower in sugar from the tables.

Talk to your dietician. Many diabetics are overwhelmed at first by the amount of knowledge required to handle their disease. Take your time. Your dietician is one of your best allies when it comes to prolonging your life.

Obese Patients

We know that exercise is an effective appetite suppressant. Studies show that obese patients move around much less each day than patients who are not obese. So, get moving. If you can't stand vigorous exercise, walk. A thirty minute walk burns off 150 calories. Since you need to burn off 3,500 calories to lose one pound, this means that, even if you eat the same amount, a daily walk will allow you to lose an extra pound of weight every twenty-three days. In other words, you'll keep off fifteen more pounds yearly if you walk than if you don't walk.

The more muscle mass you have, the more calories that you burn off even while you're sitting still. Begin a strength building program such as weight lifting. Start with a small amount of weight and increase the amount gradually. The slogan is, "Start low and go slow." See your doctor first for a good physical exam first. Then, if you have trouble motivating yourself, sign up at a health club or get a personal trainer.

Strongly restrict the *saturated* fat in your diet. This is the artery clogger that's loaded with calories. As a goal, why not aim for the same percentages of calories from fat as that found in the Japanese diet? They obtain less than ten percent of their total calories from fat and less than three per cent from saturated fat. During the three months that I live in Kobe, Japan, I rarely saw an overweight Japanese person. Eat no trans fat.

Consider drinking a glass of water before meals to obtain that comfortable full feeling before consuming as many calories. Eat slowly. Leave the table just a little bit hungry.

For your beverages, drink mostly water, tea, and skim milk. Drink the tea without cream or sugar. Since twenty percent of your daily calories come from your beverages, this is an easy way to ingest fewer calories.

Get adequate sleep. Research shows that appetite is increased significantly in people who get inadequate sleep. In addition, drowsiness has been identified as a leading cause of traffic accidents. If you're getting adequate sleep, you'll feel alert all day long. For most of us, that means eight to nine hours of sleep per night, far more than the average person gets. The body accumulates sleep debt and doesn't forget. If you've been deprived of sleep for a long time, you may need a long time to pay off that debt.

After years of treating obese patients, I feel that most patients eat to fill an emotional need. If you're unable to lose weight after an honest effort, consider seeing a therapist to discuss ways to discover and meet this need.

Hypertensive Patients

Blood pressure increases with age. Ninety percent of us will develop high blood pressure in our lives. We now rank high blood pressure as one of the most devastating health problems in terms of longevity. In other words, the higher your blood pressure is, the younger you die. So, if you want to live to a healthy old age, get your blood pressure checked regularly.

Blood pressure is "sodium sensitive" in fifty to eighty percent of patients. In other words, your blood pressure rises in proportion to the amount of salt that you eat. Consider cutting your sodium intake in half. Speak to your doctor about this.

A few suggestions may help:

First, get rid of the salt shaker at the table. If it's not there, you won't use it.

Second, don't add salt while cooking.

Third, eliminate prepared foods that are loaded with salt. Many canned soups contain 800- 900 milligrams of sodium per serving and have two servings per can. Each can of soup contains almost 2,000 milligrams of sodium. A teaspoon of table salt contains 2,300 milligrams of sodium. How many of us would add nearly a teaspoon of salt to our own bowl of soup? That's what the manufacturers regularly do.

In addition to soup, foods that promote hypertension included canned tomato products, lunch meats, and TV dinners, all loaded with salt. Be careful with salad dressing, often loaded with salt plus lots of calories from fat.

Fourth, avoid fast food restaurants. Virtually every product is loaded with salt. If you eat there, ask for a copy of their "Nutrition Facts" and check the sodium content of the food before ordering. Salads and yogurt are usually the best choices.

Low-fat dairy products may help keep blood pressure down due to their significant calcium content. Unless you can't digest milk, consume three servings of low-fat or non-fat dairy products daily. Potassium also helps to lower blood pressure. Fruits are rich in potassium.

Eat a variety of fruits daily. Diabetics should consult with a dietician before exercising this option due to the amount of sugar in fruit.

After extensive research, the United States government has published specific guidelines regarding a diet that has been shown to decrease blood pressure. They label this the DASH Eating Plan, which stands for "Dietary Approaches to Stop Hypertension." The National Heart, Lung, and Blood Institute made this plan available online at their website, www.nhlbi.nih.gov. They offer several diets, which include either 1600, 2000, 2600, or 3100 calories per day. While the best of that advice is included in this book, there is additional information available. The DASH Eating Plan is a good one.

Useful Web Sites

Many patients surf the web for information. Most often, an educated patient is a healthy patient. However, for every good web site there are ten poor ones. Many websites are slick and commercialized. Their main goal is to separate you from your money. In particular, avoid those that make outrageous claims. There is no miracle food that cures cancer, no magic diet that takes pounds off effortlessly, no mysterious supplement that provides the fountain of youth. If you're seventy-five years old now, you won't look twenty-one after using their product.

Many hucksters have their own shows on the television. Most appear on "infomercials" but others show up on "legitimate" talk shows. You'll find it far better to educate yourself.

If you do your own search on the Internet, stick with government websites or those run by well known and highly respected medical schools or hospitals. Try the following reputable sites. Remember that any site may change the look of its home page or rotate the articles that are available.

Web MD at www.webmd.com – From the home page, click on the "Eating and Diet" link of this website. There you'll find a variety of articles. Currently, the site posts a Food and Fitness Planner, a BMI Plus Calculator, and a "Food-o-Meter" which includes calorie and nutrition facts on over 37,000 foods. There are also articles on "Choosing Vitamins and Supplements" and "How to Cheat on your Diet and Still Lose Weight." The articles can change so the site may appear somewhat different. In any case, you'll find a plethora of resources.

United States Department of Agriculture at http://fnic.nal.usda. gov – These initials stand for Food and Nutrition Information Center, National Agricultural Library, United States Department of Agriculture, and, of course, government. This is the site used for nutrient counts in most of the tables in this book. From the home page, click on "Look up Calories or Nutrients in a Food." This site will be helpful if you wish to check the nutritional content of food. The tables are arranged in an easy-to-read grid format, with the foods listed in a row across the top and the nutrient values listed in a column along the left side. You'll find many similar tables in Appendix C of this book. The website also contains "Dietary Guidelines for Americans."

Center for Science in the Public Interest at www.cspinet.org – This is the website of the Center for Science in the Public Interest and the home of one of my favorite nutrition newsletters, the Nutrition Action Health Letter. The home page lists several recent articles on nutrition. You can also click on the "Ten Worst and Best Foods," or read articles on Salt, Trans Fat, and Food Dyes.

Medline Plus at www.medlineplus.gov – The National Institutes of Health, the largest medical research institute in the world, maintains this site, in conjunction with the U.S. National Library of Medicine. Here you'll have access to medical dictionaries, a medical encyclopedia, information on thousands of drugs, a directory of doctors, dentists, and hospitals, and information on local health resources, The home page features articles on 800 conditions and diseases. The site also boasts 165 interactive tutorials on a variety of medical conditions. These tutorials present slide shows with pictures and sound. If English is not your native tongue, you can also find health information in over 40 languages.

USDA Dietary Guidelines for Americans at www.health.gov/ dietaryguidelines - This government website is sponsored by the U.S. Department of Health and Human Services and the Department of Agriculture and provides quick access to the latest guidelines for healthy eating, updated every five years. The last date of issue was 2005. Guidelines for 2010 will be out soon. If you click on "Dietary

Guidelines," you can also find headings under "Weight Management," "DASH Eating Plan," "Food Safety," "Food Sources of Selected Nutrients," and "Physical Activity."

Useful Newsletters

Newsletters are a great way to keep up with the latest advice and breakthroughs on healthy eating. Most of them cost between ten and twenty dollars a year for a subscription (one to two dollars a month). This is a great bargain. You'll invariably find excellent advice every month for a minimum investment, less than a cup of java at most coffee shops. One good tip will pay you back a hundred fold in good health. A newsletter is an inexpensive way to keep abreast of developments in the field.

My favorite is *Nutrition Action Health Letter*, produced by the Center for Science in the Public Interest, a non-profit health advocacy group. Ninety percent of the content is devoted to nutrition, with an occasional article on exercise or other health concerns. They don't take advertisements. They have useful articles of general interest. The last several pages list specific foods by brand name, telling you which are healthy and which to avoid. As they say, "we name names." Speaking of nutrition newsletters, Jane Brody of the New York Times says, "My personal favorite is Nutrition Action." I agree. This newsletter is worth its weight in gold.

Consumer Reports publishes a newsletter, *On Health*, and the University of California at Berkeley publishes the *Berkeley Wellness Letter*. These last two cover many health topics including nutrition.

Most newsletters will gladly send you a free trial issue. You can easily find them online with a web search.

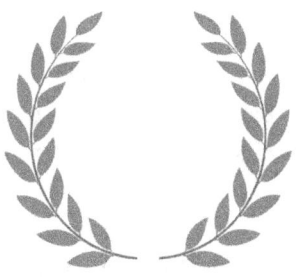

Chapter Eleven – The Final Recommendations

Twenty-Five Suggestions

If you've read the book, here's a quick summary. Or perhaps you lost interest and skipped right to this section. In either case, these are the most important recommendations in a nutshell:

1.) Eat a *wide variety* of healthy foods, especially fruits, vegetables, whole grains, peas, beans, nuts, and fish. This is the most important lesson of the book. Unless you have trouble digesting them, include three servings of low-fat dairy products daily. There is no perfect food. No one food or food group contains all the nutrients that you need.

2.) Maintain a desirable body weight your entire life.

3.) Exercise regularly. The best diet and no exercise aren't as beneficial as a good diet and regular exercise. Get twenty minutes of aerobic exercise daily. Perform strength training exercises, such as weight lifting, at least every other day. No supplement offers as much benefit as exercise. Nutrition and exercise work together like sunshine and blue skies.

4.) Eat at least three fruits a day and vary them. Eating an apple, orange, and banana every day isn't wide variety. Try papayas, cantaloupes, mangoes, apricots, prunes, kiwi, rhubarb, pineapple, and other fruits that you may not normally buy. Use your imagination.

5.) Eat at least three vegetables a day and vary them. Try asparagus, avocado, collard greens, endive, acorn squash, Brussels sprouts, kale, red peppers, and spinach. In addition, eat the common vegetables you normally find in a restaurant, such as carrots, peas, green peppers, and broccoli.

6.) Eat three or more whole grains a day. Easy choices to find in the US are oatmeal or oat bran, brown rice, sweet potato, whole wheat, and yellow corn. Vary your selection.

7.) Eat less red meat, at most three times a week. Beef, lamb, and pork are considered red meat. Choose lean meat. Beans and fish are two healthy alternatives to meat. Eat a variety of fish three times weekly.

8.) Avoid the ugly foods that are high in saturated animal fat, salt, and nitrites. These are bacon, sausage, pepperoni, salami, bologna, hot dogs, and most varieties of ham.

9.) If you don't drink alcohol, don't start. If you do drink, have at most one drink of alcohol a day. Red wine is the healthiest. If you have ever had a problem with your drinking, then don't drink any alcohol today. Your life will be fuller.

10.) If you eat a poor diet, take ONE multivitamin with minerals daily. If you're elderly, take a daily multivitamin. For men, this multivitamin shouldn't include iron. Women who are planning pregnancy or are pregnant should take a prenatal vitamin beginning four months before conception. Don't take large doses, called mega doses, of any vitamins. Even if you do take a vitamin, this doesn't replace a good diet. Nothing takes the place of eating good food. Nothing.

11.) Eat a healthy breakfast. Fruit and whole grains are a good bet. A bowl of oatmeal or multi-grain cereal is excellent. Try this healthy trio – a.) Whole grain cereal, b.) Fruit, and c.) Yogurt, skim milk, one percent milk, or organic soy milk with no added sugar.

12.) Talk to your doctor or nutritionist if you have special needs.

13.) For fluid replacement, eat fruit or drink juices from a variety of fruits. Drink several glasses of water from a good source daily. If you're not sure of its quality, have your water tested. The cost is small and may keep you from ingesting toxic or unhealthy substances. If you have a public source of drinking water, call the water department and ask them for the latest results of their mandatory testing. See how much of each pesticide, insecticide, and metal is in your water.

Chances are that the amount is extremely low in parts per billion. Tea is also an excellent drink.

14.) Read labels. Check the following items: serving size, calories, saturated fat, trans fat, cholesterol, sodium, and fiber. Watch your calories in order to maintain your ideal body weight. Avoid foods high in saturated fat and cholesterol. Eat no trans fat. Avoid foods high in sodium, especially if you have high blood pressure. Eat foods high in fiber, such as fruits, vegetables, whole grains, and beans. If a food is high in fiber, it's almost certainly good for you. Look at the first two or three ingredients on the label. These should be healthy. The first ingredients listed for many foods are often sugar, refined flour, or an unhealthy oil. Put these foods back on the shelf. Those products which contain ingredients with long, unfamiliar chemical names are highly processed foods (unless they're vitamins – learn their names). In general, the shorter that the list of ingredients is, the healthier the food is for your body. Choose ingredients with familiar, natural names, like the names of fruits, vegetables, and whole grains. Natural food was on the earth hundreds of years ago. The other 100,000 items in the grocery store are processed foods. Natural is best. Be careful with portion size. If the portion size says "two cookies" and you eat four, double all the values on the nutrition label.

15.) Keep up with the latest advice and breakthroughs on healthy eating. Subscribe to a good nutrition newsletter. My favorite is the *Nutrition Action Health Letter*, produced by the Center for Science in the Public Interest. The *Berkeley Wellness Letter* contains articles on a wide variety of health topics including nutrition.

16.) To get extra, natural vitamins, minerals, or protein into your diet, mix and make your own supplements at home. These can include a milkshake with yogurt, fruits, and nuts. As an alternative, throw several vegetables in the juicer. Use your imagination. This will be far healthier than any energy bar you can purchase.

17.) Instead of the grocery, try shopping at a health food store or your local outdoor market.

18.) Instead of the usual fast food restaurant, try a vegetarian restaurant.

19.) Buy a heart healthy cook book.

20.) Slow down. Take your time. Savor your food. Share your meal with someone you love.

21.) Get adequate sleep. People who are tired eat more than those who get adequate sleep. If you're getting adequate sleep, you'll feel alert all day long.

22.) If you smoke, quit. If you don't smoke, don't start.

23.) Learn how to handle stress before stress manhandles you. The best methods are meditation, yoga, exercise, and proper breathing. Physicians and researchers at Harvard University have extensively studied the effects of transcendental meditation and confirmed its benefits in lowering blood pressure, heart rate, respiratory rate, and oxygen consumption. Visit your local library and borrow the book *The Relaxation Response* by Herbert Benson, M.D.

24.) If you don't have time to read a book on relaxation, learn diaphragmatic breathing. Take ten deep diaphragmatic breaths at least three times daily. Research shows that proper breathing has a multitude of beneficial effects, from decreasing stress to minimizing hot flashes.

25.) If all else fails, read the next section on the art of nutrition.

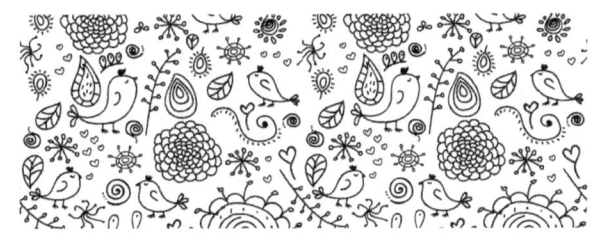

Chapter Twelve - The Art of Nutrition

We've talked a lot about the science of nutrition and the proper foods to eat. You may find some of this a bit dry and boring. Is there an art to nutrition? In other words, now that we know *what* to eat, should we also know *how* to eat? Are there ways to amplify the benefits of eating healthy foods? Of course there are.

Improve All Four Phases of Nutrition

We previously learned about the four phases of nutrition: ingestion, digestion, metabolism, and elimination. The first phase, ingestion, has been the major focus so far. When we choose nutritious food meal after meal, day after day, we put into effect powerful changes that will enable us to have strong, healthy bodies for many years. Unless you're in a prison camp or a hospital, you have some control over the food you choose. Use the power wisely. However, don't force yourself to eat foods you dislike. Instead, improve your mood and attitude by choosing healthy foods that you really love.

Three other hints will help you choose wisely. First, remember that portion size is crucial. You can greatly decrease calories and weight gain simply by eating smaller portions. Second, be aware of the content of your food. Know what you're eating. Third, be mindful while eating.

Would you like to do a fun experiment? The next time you're at the movie theatre, watch the food that people choose at the snack bar. Often, they'll choose a "super maximum gigantic gulp," a soft drink containing far more fluid than their bladder capacity, plus an appropriately named "tub" of popcorn far bigger than their head.

It's simple but elementary - bigger portions contain more calories.

One frequent bit of advice for obese patients is simply to decrease portion size. Another is to put the same amount of food on a smaller plate. People who do so eat less.

As the Zen master would say, "Only eat to satisfy your need, not to excess."

Next, know the content of all food that you put into your mouth. The movie goers who choose popcorn inadvertently consume mountains of calories and fat, since the popcorn in movie theatres is often cooked with palm or coconut oils. The helpful employee behind the counter then asks, "Would you like butter with that?" and, after receiving an affirmative answer, covers this with melted butter out of a faucet. A large tub of movie theatre popcorn cooked in coconut oil contains 1,100 calories. If you add butter, the tub contains 1,600 calories. Perhaps we should call this monstrosity the "cruise missile of calories." Eat one bucket and your waist line explodes.

As the Zen master would say, "Attention. Attention. Pay attention."

On top of this, many people watching the movie don't even taste the food they're eating, since their attention is focused on the film. If they are going to expand their waist line, they should at least enjoy the process. Eating during any other activity detracts from the pleasure of eating. So, don't eat while you're driving, reading, watching a movie, or even having sex, for that matter. Don't eat while engaged in other activities. Be mindful.

As the Zen master would say, "When you eat, just eat."

The second phase, digestion, is also important. Some advocates of red wine feel that a small glass with the evening meal provides a bit of tranquility. Tea drinkers claim an improved digestion with certain varieties, most commonly peppermint or green tea. Many restaurants play soothing background music while their guests eat.

A simple way you can improve your digestion is by chewing your food well. John D. Rockefeller, Sr., the founder of Standard Oil and an American business tycoon, lived from 1839 to 1937. In the early 1900s, he announced that he would live to be one hundred years old. One of the means by which he chose to reach this goal was to chew his food well. He chewed each bite at least ten times. Guests who came to visit him finished their own lunch and then got to sit and watch

John D. take almost another hour. That's how long he took to eat his food, always. He lived to be almost ninety-eight during an era when the average life expectancy was forty-seven.

So, eat slowly. Chew your food well. Remain calm and relaxed while eating. Maintain a tranquil mind and spirit. Background music, a glass of wine, or a cup of tea may add to the atmosphere of tranquility. Remember that you're now eating healthy, nutritious, natural food that will vitalize your body. So, taste each bite. Savor your food. Don't gulp. Chew slowly until your food is easy to swallow. Slow down and eat your food mindfully. Really enjoy eating.

The third phase is metabolism. By getting the necessary amounts of all the micronutrients that our bodies require to facilitate chemical reactions, we can improve our metabolism. These nutrients are vitamins and minerals. Our metabolism is helped by getting adequate sleep, exercising, avoiding stress, and not smoking.

The fourth phase is elimination. Eating adequate fiber aids in the transit of food along the GI tract. Exercise helps to stimulate adequate peristalsis, the rhythmic movement of the intestines. Drink adequate water and other fluids to enable your body to rid itself of the toxins that all food produces, such as the nitrogenous byproducts of protein that we eliminate through urination. Promptly eliminate waste (go to the bathroom) when the call arises. Don't wait for hours to honor nature, as many children and even some adults do. Get this priority straight. Listen to Nature's call, stop the car if necessary, and hit the rest room.

Eat Happy, Healthy Food

If you're a picky eater and won't change your habits, choose several healthy foods that you love. Eat lots of those. This is particularly helpful if you don't have the time or motivation to follow the suggestions to eat a wide variety of foods. The Greek and Japanese diets often contain the same healthy foods every day. For example, the Japanese diet contains lots of fish, rice, local vegetables, and green tea. The people eat these every day for years.

When I lived in Mexico, I saw many poor Mexican families eat rice and beans every day with whatever vegetables were available.

Occasionally they had chicken. This is a healthy diet. Rice and beans together contain all of the essential amino acids. The so-called Mexican food that we eat in the US is loaded with sour cream, cheese, and, pureed fried beans, called frijoles, that often contain lard. Instead, eat a genuine Mexican diet with lots of whole beans, whole grain rice, lean chicken, and vegetables. Finish with a little fruit. That's an excellent meal.

To eat food that makes us happy is good.

To eat food that makes us healthy is better.

To eat food that makes us happy and healthy is best.

Cheat a Little

Do I have any more ideas for eating well? You may want to cheat on your diet.

Cheat?

That's right. Cheat.

The famous psychotherapist Milton Erickson once treated a patient who had tried everything to lose weight. She would lose weight for a while and then rebound, gaining back even more than she lost. Further questioning revealed that the client would follow her diet faithfully for a few weeks. Then she would start eating voraciously. Once she fell back into this habit, she was unable to control her consumption and would binge for several weeks. Her weight would skyrocket.

Erickson struck a deal with his patient. They agreed that she would watch her diet carefully for three weeks. Then, on the Sunday of the third week, she would eat whatever she wanted, all day long. Knowing that she could binge, the woman watched her diet carefully for three weeks. Then, on the day she was allowed to binge with the doctor's permission, she did eat what she wanted, but found that she didn't eat as much as on an average day of cheating before this agreement. On Monday morning, she went back to her regular diet for another three weeks. The result was a consistent, significant amount of weight loss.

As Bernie Siegel says, "I've done the research, and I hate to tell you, but everybody dies – lovers, joggers, vegetarians, and non-smokers. I'm telling you this so that some of you who jog at five a.m. and eat vegetables will occasionally sleep late and have an ice cream cone."[1]

So, since you're going to die anyway, why not cheat a little bit? Give yourself a set amount of time to binge, whether for one meal, one day, or whatever. Decide when and how much you will cheat before you go hog wild.

Then, enjoy the food. Savor that trip to the fast food restaurant, that huge banana split, that piece of pie with ice cream. Everyone has a favorite bad food. If you can't live without bacon, allow yourself a big Sunday breakfast with bacon.

I've never had any patient stick to a strict diet for long without cheating. Many are so strict with themselves that, when they come crashing off their diet, they eat like a starving person for days, regaining much of the lost weight. It's better to knowingly eat a cheeseburger once a week than to sneak one every day, pretending that you're not. The important thing is to give yourself permission to eat those delicious but unhealthy foods, restricting this activity to specific times and amounts. Enjoy them. Then, get back to eating healthily. Allowing yourself an occasional lapse will help you to stick to your plan. And you will find it easier to stay on your diet knowing that you can look forward to a break.

Learn to control your cheating rather than letting your cheating control you.

Eat in Gratitude

According to commonly accepted statistics, one-fourth of the world's population goes to bed hungry every night. Since there are six billion people on the Earth, one and a half billion go to bed hungry. Incredibly, as many as 20,000 children in the undeveloped Third World die of starvation every day, most of them in Africa.

Meanwhile, in the developed civilizations, our markets and grocery stores carry an incredible array of food. The amount and variety of food is astronomical: meat, poultry, and fish; a huge variety of fruits and vegetables, fresh, frozen, and canned; potatoes, rice, wheat, corn, oats, and a harvest of exotic grains; cereals, breads, bagels, pasta, cakes, cookies, pies, crackers, corn chips, pretzels; milk, cheese butter,

---

[1]Siegel, Bernie, M.D. Peace, Love, and Healing. Harper Collins.

ice cream, yogurt, and eggs; juices, coffee, tea, wine, and beer. On any given day, there may be over one hundred brands of breakfast cereal in the average grocery store. We have a wealth of food to choose from that is many times greater than the choice of even the richest of kings or emperors in the Middle Ages. Charlemagne would have marveled at one trip to a grocery store. Many of these items end up on the home pantry shelf; yet how often do we go to the cupboard, looking for food, only to say, "There's nothing to eat." Meanwhile, thousands of children continue to die of starvation every day.

To take a new perspective, consider the following. Let's say that your breakfast consists of orange juice or tea, milk and cereal, eggs, toast and jelly. Let's consider the orange juice, which likely came from Florida or California. Someone planted the orange trees years ago, then watered, fertilized, and cultivated them until the fruit was mature. A group of workers, often underpaid, spent hours in the sun picking the oranges. Another group transported the fruit to the factory, where it was washed, peeled, and squeezed into cardboard containers that were made at yet another factory. The juice was transported in a refrigerated truck, itself a marvel of manufacturing. A truck driver drove the juice a thousand miles to a warehouse in your city, where it was distributed to the supermarket near your home where another worker unpacked and placed it on the shelf. You spend your three dollars to buy it, perhaps complaining about the price, as yet another worker, the cashier, rings up the sale.

The tea came from China or India, since our northern climate is not favorable to its growth and cultivation. You would have a long boat ride or a very long swim if you obtained the tea yourself. A laborer was paid the equivalent of a few pennies a day to tend and harvest the tea. The tea leaves were then sent to a factory where they were prepared and packaged in bulk, delivered by truck to an ocean going vessel, and shipped thousands of miles across a sometimes treacherous ocean to the shores of your country. There someone packaged the tea into individual packets so that you could dip a single tea bag into your morning cup. Similarly, if you drink coffee, the beans were planted, grown, cultivated, and picked in South America, then went through a similar labor-intensive process to arrive at your local grocery store.

The water in your cup was pumped from a local lake, tested for dozens of toxic substances, filtered to remove any debris or sediment, and chlorinated to remove pathogens. The cup itself may have been hand made and painted in yet another country, then packed and transported to a warehouse, then packaged, shipped overseas, unloaded, and sent to a merchant in a retail store who displays and then sells the cup to you.

The eggs probably came from a local farm. The farmer cared for the chickens from the day that they were hatched, giving them food, water, and shelter, cleaning their cages, giving immunizations, and collecting the eggs. These eggs were then shipped to a factory to be cleaned, packaged, and transported in another truck to your supermarket.

The grain for your toast or cereal was grown at yet another farm, or probably several farms, then prepared and transported. The sugar in your jelly may have come from sugar cane in Florida, sugar beets in Utah, or perhaps from a foreign country. The fruit in your jelly came from yet another farm and was prepared and packaged in yet another factory.

You prepare your toast in an electric toaster, which cost twenty dollars at a local department store. Yet this toaster took hundreds of people working together in a factory to assemble it from dozens of raw materials, which were mined and collected in different parts of the world. The stove on which you cook your eggs came from yet another factory. The power to provide the electricity to prepare your meal on the stove came from Midwestern coal transported hundreds of miles by train. Or perhaps, if you use a gas range, the energy came from Middle Eastern oil, transported thousands of miles by ship to our shores, refined, transported, and converted to a form of fuel that you can use in your home.

When we think of the process, having a simple breakfast at home may not seem so ordinary anymore. If we keep a gratitude journal, having breakfast could count as one entry for the day. Then again, each food that we eat, whether toast, eggs, or jelly, each appliance that we use, the refrigerator, toaster, stove, and coffee maker, and each item of tableware, the plate, cup, or spoon, could count as one item. At the end of breakfast, we have a new appreciation for the dozens of products and thousands of people who enrich our lives daily. When we look at our world in this way, every meal becomes an occasion of gratitude and a source of wonder.

Behind the simple loaf of bread sitting on the breakfast table lie so many miracles, people, and stories. A small seed planted in the brown earth grows into a mature plant. The laborer in the field carefully cultivates the harvest. Hundreds of hands transport each product every step of the way. Finally, someone prepares this food with loving kindness. Once we truly see this, we can appreciate our daily bread in a more profound way.

Perhaps this is another reason why people who eat breakfast live longer, fuller lives.

An Oasis of Peace

One of the busiest times of my life was my three-year residency in family medicine. I worked as many as one hundred hours a week. I was on call every four days for three years. Our regular shift was 7 a.m. to 5 p.m. Being on call meant being there all night in addition to our regular hours. For example, if I was on call on Monday, I entered the hospital at 8 a.m. on Monday and left at 5 p.m. on Tuesday evening. Since call occurred every four days, the process repeated itself on Friday, with the exception that I could leave at noon on Saturday. When we were on call, we never knew how much sleep we would get, if any.

There were always more patients to see, more labs to check, more babies to deliver, more lectures to attend. I rushed constantly, didn't get enough sleep, and ate whatever the hospital cafeteria provided. Back then, nutrition wasn't taught in medical school. In fact, no one knew much about nutrition, so most of the cafeteria food was less than optimal. Since the hospital provided all of our meals for free while we were working, I ate every lunch and dinner there, Monday through Friday, and weekends too, if I was on call. If "you are what you eat," then, for good or for bad, after three years of residency, I was a walking glob of hospital food.

In spite of the great number of factors beyond my control during this time, I did one thing well. I gave myself a half an hour to eat. No matter how many sick patients we had on the floors, I gave myself permission to eat my meal slowly and calmly. Often, without knowing it, I would assume the lotus position while seated at the table. I had both legs crossed over each other, on top of my chair seat, each foot resting on the opposite thigh, under the table. I hoped that I wasn't noticed, since this wasn't considered a proper way to sit. As a child in a restaurant, if I'd sat this way, my mother may have told me to put my feet on the floor.

I ate slowly and took time to let my food digest, no matter how busy the day, no matter how much work remained to be done. This became my *one* time not to hurry. The doctors had a separate dining room, so I also enjoyed the company of several colleagues during this time, as we sat together in a group at a large round table.

One day a fellow resident, a physician from India, noticed that I sat in the lotus position and asked me why I sat like that. I told him that I sat this way automatically, without thinking, because it was comfortable and allowed me to slow down mentally. He told me that many people in his country sat this way but that he had never seen an American do so in public. He seemed genuinely pleased to see me eat this way, perhaps since I reminded him of his homeland. For me, it was a matter of habit, comfort, and relaxation. My body was more limber, the hips, pelvis, and spine suppler, my stomach muscles more relaxed, my legs more comfortable. I felt calmer.

In my mind, eating lunch in that hectic hospital became associated with an attitude of not hurrying, of taking my time, of eating deliberately. Sitting in the lotus position helped me to create an oasis of serenity in a desert of hurry and stress. To use a modern psychological term, the physical alignment of my body became a kinesthetic *anchor* for feelings of relaxation and tranquility that I experienced every time I sat this way.

Perhaps another story will prove interesting. My friend Tom told me about his Grandfather Ivan. For years, the man disregarded two of the rules of good health – eating properly and getting regular exercise. When he was young, Tom often spent weekends with Grandpa Ivan and his family. For Grandpa Ivan, Sunday breakfast consisted of two fried eggs and several strips of bacon, followed by half a dozen donuts, all washed down with a couple glasses of whole milk. The family then sat around for hours playing Risk®. For lunch, they usually polished off the donuts and continued playing.

This same grandfather worked a desk job for years. When he received a nice promotion with more responsibility, he lasted one month before choosing to return to his old job with less pay and less stress. He said that he didn't want more responsibility. He also didn't care about the pay raise since his needs were simple.

He retired as young as possible and now spends most of his time watching sports on television. Grandpa Ivan's main form of exercise is to walk from the television to the refrigerator. He often brags to people that he "loves to do nothing better than anything." He's married to a wife who is described as extremely difficult. Yet he never seems ruffled by anything that she says or does, choosing to ignore virtually all of her behavior. They have seven children, most of whom work in mundane jobs, none of whom completed college. He would never be described as having a Type A personality.

As far as good habits, he doesn't smoke or drink alcohol. He occasionally takes an evening walk. His weight has always been near ideal. In fact, he was often referred to as "a tall drink of water" or "skinny as a bean pole." Now seventy years old, he has had no health problems.

His life is incredibly free of stress. The one time he experienced tension, in his new job, he quickly gave up the promotion and extra pay to return to his old position.

What lesson can we derive from good old Grandpa Ivan? Well, perhaps peace of mind may be as important as what we eat. So, if you choose not to eat well, then work to become the most relaxed person on earth.

Allow me to relate another story. During medical school, a group of students spent a day in the hospital with a cardiologist from Venezuela named Luis. This doctor was your typical "jolly fat person." When we went on rounds, he seemed to know everyone that we passed. He always said hello and usually had a joke or two. When we passed a nurse in the hallway who was obviously pregnant, he asked, "Are you pregnant AGAIN?" "Yes, I am," she replied. "Which one is this?" he asked. "This will be my eighth child," she replied." "My God, you haven't had a period in the seven years you've been married, have you?" he asked, smiling. "Yes, a couple," she replied, laughing, "and I've been married for eleven years. Haven't you been putting on a little weight?"

Unlike the other physicians who wore long white coats as a symbol of their authority, Luis wore a blue coat, similar to the ones worn by workers at the local grocery named Farmer Jack's. When another physician passed us in the hall, he said to Luis, "Are you still wearing that butcher's coat from Farmer Jack's?" "Yes, I am," said Louis. "They don't pay me enough here so I moonlight there at night. It's cheaper just to wear this coat to my second job." The two physicians then engaged in a round of good-natured banter, obviously enjoying each other's company. Doctor Luis seemed to interact like this with everyone that we passed. He was a pleasure to spend time with. I don't recall meeting another doctor like him during four years of medical school and three years of residency. Many doctors seem to lose the joy of life, along with their sense of humor, never to find them again.

After rounds, we went to his office to discuss the cases we had seen on the cardiology wards. At that time, most heart attack patients were men. Doctor Luis asked us what caused these attacks. We spewed out the usual possibilities, including hypertension, a high fat diet, smoking, and so on. His answer was interesting. He said, "Here, heart attacks are very common. We see them all the time. When I was a medical student in Venezuela, a heart attack was so rare that, when a patient was admitted to the hospital with one, all the medical students scrambled to see him. You know, the people in Venezuela eat as much fatty food as here, lots of butter, cream, and meat. They smoke just as much, probably more. I think what causes heart attacks is the stress. Everyone here is in a hurry. That stress will kill you."

I read in the National Geographic magazine of a man in India who is a bit unusual. He hasn't worn clothes in forty-six years, choosing to be naked. He spends much of his time meditating. What does this have to do with nutrition? Well, he reportedly eats only a glass of milk and a banana daily. He's practiced this lifestyle for nearly half a century and claims to have no medical problems. I'm not sure if this character occasionally sneaks other food or even if he takes a daily multivitamin.

Admittedly, his nutritional needs are small and his stress level must be one of the lowest in the world. He may not accomplish a lot by Western standards. We know that milk contains a great variety of nutrients. But his culinary habits go against all the recommendations about eating a wide variety of healthy foods. So, he should not thrive on this restricted diet.

I confess that the man puzzles me. I can only attempt to answer this nutritional conundrum. Perhaps, if you put yourself in an extremely meditative state of mind, lower your energy requirements drastically, and live a stress-free life, you can survive on a meager diet. Or perhaps he's engaging in a little bragging and secretly eats more than he claims. It's certainly food for thought.

I believe that the best advice is to eat a balanced, nutritious diet *and* to lead a life as free of stress as reasonably possible.

You too can find an anchor to slow yourself down while you eat your meal, no matter how little time you have or how stressful your occupation. You can use a prayer before meals, the lotus sitting position, calming music, a favorite meal partner. Any behavior that anchors a feeling of peace can serve this purpose. I believe that this practice will pay rewards in calming your spirit and aiding your digestion, allowing you to absorb your food well and to metabolize the nutrients properly.

Make the meal time an oasis of calm and tranquility in your daily life, even if the rest of your life is in disarray. Don't eat when you are angry, hurried, or worried. Come to the table with a clear mind and a peaceful heart. Choose to share your food with those you love, in whose company you find yourself relaxed.

You may wish to prepare a healthy meal for yourself and your family. Even if you don't like to cook, making a meal with family or friends can turn a chore into an enjoyable activity. Make the atmosphere in your kitchen as tranquil as possible. Create an ambience that is conducive to a delicious and hearty meal. Then eat mindfully, really tasting your food, savoring each bite. Being calm and mindful will enable you to enjoy each meal more and to eagerly anticipate the next repast.

Most of all, don't rush your food. Someone once wrote that stress is the feeling of not having enough time. If only one activity of your day can be restful, make it every mealtime. Allow this to be *your* time. Separate yourself from negative emotions such as anger, greed, fear, and worry. Even if you normally rush all day, in fact, especially if you rush all day, let your meal be an island of unhurried tranquility in the chaotic sea of life.

Visualize

Not only is it helpful to eat mindfully, but we can use visualization to aid digestion.

As you eat, chew each mouthful slowly and mindfully. Taste your food. After you chew well and swallow, picture the food entering your stomach and small intestines, where it is gently broken down by the digestive enzymes. Then, visualize the food entering your clear bloodstream, free of obstruction, where the nutrients are picked up by healthy carrier proteins and transported to all the appropriate organs: the carbohydrates to the liver, the glucose to the brain, and the proteins to the muscles.

See each organ or tissue in turn becoming healthy, invigorated, and vital. Picture the muscles in your body growing powerful and flexible. See your bones becoming sturdy and strong. Imagine your brain receiving the proper amounts of oxygen and glucose. Picture the individual cells receiving their microscopic amount of nutrient broth, invigorating the mitochondria, the little factories that produce prodigious amounts of energy. If you're injured, see the broken bone or laceration receiving its share of healthy nutrients and undergoing the process of proper healing. If you're ill, notice the nutrient-rich blood delivering a care package to the affected body part, whether it is the ulcer in your stomach, the infection in your sinuses, or the cut on your skin. Relax and breathe peacefully while performing this visualization.

Companionship, Love, Touching

Adding some love, companionship, or friendship in your day, whether you have to beg, borrow, or bribe to get it, pays rich rewards to your health and peace of mind. Recently, my priest spoke about nutrition during a sermon that he gave on the subject of love. He mentioned studies showing that rabbits fed a junk food diet but given lots of stroking and attention, outlived rabbits that were given a healthy diet and no love.

He was probably referring to a study done at Ohio University in the 1970s. The researchers fed a high-cholesterol diet to a group of rabbits and found damage to the arteries in all groups except one, which surprisingly showed few symptoms even though they were fed the same toxic diet. Later, it was discovered that the student in charge of this group of rabbits used to lovingly hold, pet, and fondle the rabbits in the bottom row of cages before feeding them. These rabbits showed few signs of damaged arteries. The rabbits in the higher cages that the student couldn't reach didn't receive the affection. Similar results were found in later experiments when one group of rabbits received lots of stroking while the others were treated neutrally.

The obvious conclusion is that, when a rabbit is loved, or at least petted fondly, its entire body functions better. In another study, researchers observed people from different cultures during an hour of conversation to see how often they touched. People from the "warmer" Mediterranean and Latin cultures touched over one hundred times per hour. People from the colder, northern cultures touched from zero to four times per hour. Perhaps another reason why the people in Luis' home country of Venezuela suffered fewer heart attacks is greater frequency of human touch.

When we find love, we discover a higher purpose for ourselves than our own little bag of needs and wants. I am convinced that one reason there are so many shelves of self-help books in the United States is because so many people feel unloved in a society that puts its greatest emphasis on career, money, and material possessions.

The healthiest rabbits and people are probably those that eat a good diet and are loved too.

In another study, premature babies in the Neonatal Intensive Care Unit of a hospital were separated into two groups. Both groups had their basic needs fulfilled. However, the babies in the second group were caressed three times a day for twenty minutes by volunteers, usually senior citizens, who had received special training in how to stroke the babies for this study.

What do you think happened?

The study had to be called off long before it had run its proposed course. Researchers felt it was unethical and medically unsound to continue. The babies in the control group, who had their basic needs for survival met but were not stroked, were dying at a much higher rate than the babies who were touched. The ramifications of this study are profound. As early as birth, even if it occurs weeks or months prematurely, we cannot survive without love. Perhaps the smallest human beings can teach us what the wisest adults have forgotten.

When we're touched or stroked several times a day, we thrive and grow.

So, why not share your meal with someone you love, even if your meal is just bread and fruit from the local market? Sitting on a blanket in the sunshine on a warm summer day is a pleasant way to share a meal. Engage in conversation or share the intimacy of silence. Touch each other frequently. Give each other a massage afterward. Then go for a walk. Or, if the weather is inclement, share a bath together. Or listen to music. Or….use your imagination.

Learn Two Sentences to Survive

If you've learned to love, you've learned an even more valuable lesson than that of good nutrition. As Louis L'Amour said in his book, *The Walking Drum*, "It has occurred to me that a man need know but two sentences to survive. The first to ask for food, the second to tell a woman he loves her. If he must dispense with one or the other, by all means let it be the first – for surely, if you tell a woman you love her, she will feed you."[2]

May you grow healthy and strong. May you surround yourself with love. May the food you consume nourish you properly for many long, enjoyable years. As the Vulcans say, "May you live long and prosper."

Here's to your health.

---

[2] L'Amour, Louis. The Walking Drum. 1984. Bantam Books.

Appendices

Appendix A – Simple Sample Menu Plan

BREAKFAST

1.) Choose one of the following (½ - ¾ cup):
> Oatmeal
> Whole grain oat cereal
> Whole grain corn cereal
> Multigrain cereal with all whole grains, or
> Whole grain toast or bagel

2.) Plus one of the following (½ – ¾ cup):
> Blueberries
> Blackberries
> Raspberries
> Strawberries
> Or other healthy fruits, preferably a variety

3.) Choose one of the following (4 – 8 ounces):
> Skim or 1% milk, or,
> Yogurt, 4 ounces
> Soy milk if you are lactose intolerant

4.) Optionally, add one of the following (one tablespoon or ten nuts):
> Almonds, walnuts, or pecans

OR, as an alternative breakfast, choose the following once or twice a week:

> 2 – 3 medium boiled eggs or egg whites (the yolk contains all the cholesterol and most of the vitamins. Substitute egg whites on

your physician's advice)
    Beans of your choice (see "Great Beans")
    Whole corn tortilla
    Fresh fruit

LUNCH

1.) Choose one of the following:
    Vegetable soup, 1 cup
    Vegetable medley, fresh or frozen, gently steam or microwave,
    ½ - 1 cup
    Salad with healthy lettuce and fresh vegetables, 1 cup
    Note #1: For optional dressing, use vinegar and olive oil or 1-2
        tablespoons of light salad dressing with no more than 6
        grams of fat, all unsaturated.
    Note #2: Regarding "healthy lettuce," iceberg lettuce is mostly
        water. While it adds minimal calories, there are few nutri-
        ents other than a small amount of Vitamin K. More nutri-
        tious choices include romaine, red leaf, or bib lettuce which
        are easily accessible in the grocery store. Turnip or collard
        greens are also healthy, but should be cooked with onions,
        green pepper, or lean chicken, not with salt pork, bacon, or
        ham hocks. For the ambitious, bok choy and Swiss chard
        are great choices and can be stir fried with a small amount
        of healthy oil.

2.) Add one of the following:
    Whole wheat bread, 1-2 slices, 2-3 grams of fiber per slice
    (One slice of regular bread or 2 slices of light bread contain
    about 40 calories)
    Whole grain crackers

3.) Add one of the following:
    One slice of low fat cheese (Part-skim milk cheese contains
    less than 5 grams of fat per ounce)
    Tofu
    Soy beans
    Low-fat cottage cheese

4.) As an option, or on strenuous days, add 3-4 ounces:

Tuna (chunk light preferred to albacore)
Sardines
Lunch meat (lean chicken or turkey)
Lean beef
Optional dessert: 1-2 whole grain cookies with no trans fat.

DINNER

1.) Choose one of the following healthy carbohydrates:
Yams, ½ cup
Sweet potatoes, ½ cup
Squash, acorn or butternut, 1 cup
Whole grain brown rice, ½ - ¾ cup
Barley, ½ - ¾ cup
Occasionally, a "starchy" vegetable, such as peas, corn, or lima
beans, ½ cup

2.) Add one vegetable from each of the following rows:
Broccoli, cabbage, cauliflower, Brussels sprouts
Red or yellow peppers
Carrots, eggplant, okra, spinach, leafy or turnip greens
prepared with no meat
Zucchini, asparagus, plain beets, green or wax beans,
summer squash (less starchy than acorn or butternut)
Tomato
Alternatively, make a healthy salad with mixed greens and a
rainbow of vegetables.

3.) Add your bean of choice (½ cup):
Black
Garbanzo (chick peas)
Kidney
Navy
Pinto
White
Lentils

4.) OR, alternate your bean of choice with fish (4 – 8 ounces) two to
three times a week:
Flounder

Salmon, wild

Trout

Other fish without the skin

OR, once or twice a week, if preferred, substitute one of the following meats for the fish or beans:

Turkey or chicken, skinless, mostly white meat, no organ meat (liver, kidney)

Lean beef

SNACKS

Choose one of the following for a mid-morning or mid-afternoon snack:

1.) Variety of colorful fruits (the portion is a small tennis ball size or ½ cup, except for berries and melon, when up to 1 cup may be eaten)

2.) Variety of nuts, favoring almonds and walnuts, also pecans, cashews, pistachios

(¼ cup, unsalted)

3.) Pumpkin or sunflower seeds, unsalted, ½ cup

4.) Low-fat yogurt or cottage cheese, ½ cup

5.) Fresh vegetables, ½ - 1 cup, with low-fat dip, if preferred

6.) Whole grain cereal (1 slice), or 1 slice of toast with small amount of honey

7.) Whole grain chips, 1 ounce, with garden salsa containing tomatoes, corn, and beans, ¼ cup

8.) Whole grain pretzels, 1 ounce

9.) Light popcorn, 1 serving with less than 3 grams of fat, no trans fat

10.) Power drink with low-fat yogurt, fruit, and nuts whipped up in a blender.

BEVERAGES

Free beverages (considered to contain minimal to no calories) include the following:

1.) Vegetable juices, no salt, ½ cup
2.) Herbal tea, green tea, or black tea, unsweetened
3.) Water, 8 – 12 ounces

Note: The first three are preferred beverages.

4.) Coffee, unsweetened, with 1 TBSP skim milk if preferred
5.) Diet soda or sugar-free beverage, 8 – 12 ounces

Other healthy beverages containing calories:

1.) Fruit juices with the pulp, ½ cup or four ounces
2.) Skim milk (80 calories per cup)
3.) Soy milk, plain (70 – 100 calories per cup)
4.) Rice milk, unflavored (70 – 100 calories per cup)

Note: Flavored soy milk or rice milk contain 160 – 200 calories per cup.

5.) Red wine, 4 ounces

Appendix B – Equivalent Measurements, Metric and Conventional

¼ cup = 2 fluid ounces = 4 tablespoons
½ cup = 4 fluid ounces = 8 tablespoons
1 cup = 8 ounces = 16 tablespoons
1 gallon = 4 quarts = 8 pints = 16 cups = 128 ounces
1 ounce = 28 grams
3.5 ounces = 100 grams

Appendix C – Tables of Nutrient Values

As with all such tables in this book, the food is arranged by category – nuts, meats, fruits, vegetables, and so on. The food is listed horizontally across the top row. The nutrients are listed along the left hand column. These include water, calories, protein, fat, carbohydrate, fiber, sugars, and many vitamins and minerals. Farther down the table are the values for saturated fat and cholesterol.

All values are from the United States Department of Agriculture, which has been collecting data on food content for over one hundred years. Their web site, www.nal.usda.gov/fnic/foodcomp, contains the nutrient values for over ten thousand foods, some by brand name. The order for the nutrients on the left hand side of the tables in this book is the same as that found on the web site, which is even more complete, containing a breakdown of fatty acids and proteins. If a nutrient isn't listed on the left hand side of the table, the food doesn't contain it. (For example, Vitamin D is often omitted from the left hand column). Remember that Vitamin D can be elusive during the winter months and Vitamin B_{12} is not found in a vegetarian diet.

Unless otherwise noted, all values are for 100 grams of the edible portion of the food. 100 grams is equal to three and one-half ounces. If you eat more or less, adjust the values for the nutrients appropriately. For example, if you eat seven ounces, double all the values.

NUTS	Almond	Cashew	Hazelnut	Macadamia	Peanut	Pecan	Pistachio	Walnut
Water (g)	5.25	5.20	5.31	1.36	6.50	3.52	3.97	4.56
Energy (Kcal)	578	566	628	718	567	691	557	618
Protein (g)	21.26	18.22	14.95	7.91	25.80	9.17	20.61	24.06
Total Fat (g)	50.64	46.92	60.75	75.77	49.24	71.97	44.44	59.0
Carbohy-drates (g)	19.74	27.13	16.70	13.82	16.13	13.86	27.97	9.91
Fiber (g)	11.8	3.3	9.7	8.6	8.5	9.6	10.3	6.8
Sugars, total (g)	4.80	5.91	4.34	4.57	3.97	3.97	7.64	1.10
Calcium (mg)	248	37	114	85	92	70	107	61
Iron (mg)	4.30	6.68	4.7	3.69	4.58	2.53	4.15	3.12
Magnesium (mg)	275	292	163	130	168	121	121	201
Phosphorus (mg)	474	593	290	188	376	277	490	513
Potassium (mg)	728	660	680	368	705	410	1025	523
Sodium (mg)	1	12	0	5	18	0	1	2
Zinc (mg)	3.36	5.78	2.45	1.3	3.27	4.53	2.2	3.37

NUTS	Almond	Cashew	Hazelnut	Macadamia	Peanut	Pecan	Pistachio	Walnut
Copper (mg)	1.110	2.195	1.725	0.756	1.144	1.20	1.3	1.36
Manganese (mg)	2.535	1.655	6.175	4.131	1.934	4.50	1.2	3.896
Selenium (mcg)	2.8	19.9	2.4	3.6	7.2	3.8	7.0	17.0
Vitamin C (mg)	0.0	0.5	6.3	1.2	0.0	1.1	5.0	1.7
Thiamin (mg)	0.241	0.423	0.643	1.195	0.640	0.660	0.87	0.057
Riboflavin (mg)	0.811	0.058	0.113	0.162	0.135	0.130	0.16	0.13
Niacin (mg)	3.925	1.062	1.800	2.473	12.066	1.167	1.30	0.47
Pantothenic acid (mg)	0.349	0.864	0.918	0.758	1.767	0.863	0.520	1.660
Vitamin B-6 (mg)	0.131	0.417	0.563	0.275	0.348	0.210	1.7	0.583
Folate (mcg)	29	25	113	11	240	22	51	31
B-12 (mcg)	0.0	0.00	0.00	0.0	0.0	0.0	0.0	0.0
Vitamin A (IU)	5	0	20	0	0.0	56	553	40
Vitamin E (mg)	25.87	0.9	15.03	0.54	8.33	1.40	2.30	1.8
Vitamin K (mcg)	0.0	34.1	14.2	0	0.0	3.5	0	2.7
Saturated Fat (g)	3.881	8.328	4.464	12.06	6.834	6.18	5.44	3.368
Cholesterol (mg)	0	0	0	0	0	0	0	0
Beta Carotene (mcg)	3	0	11	0	0	29	332	24
Alpha Carotene (mcg)	0	0	3	0	0	0	0	0

All values are per 100 grams, about 2/3 of a cup.

Here are some thoughts on the table. A 100 gram portion is about two-thirds of a cup, a sizeable amount. Nuts are high in fat, mostly unsaturated, although cashews and macadamia nuts have more saturated fat, almonds and walnuts, less. Nuts are rich in calcium, iron, magnesium, phosphorous, potassium, zinc, and manganese, along with some selenium, copper and niacin. Almonds are high in Vitamin E, cashews in Vitamin K, and pistachios in Vitamin A. None contain Vitamin B_{12} or Vitamin D.

MEAT	Bacon, raw	Bacon, broiled or fried	Beef, Ground, Broiled	Bologna, Pork	Chicken, meat & skin, roasted	Lamb	Pepperoni, pork, beef	Sausage, Pork, cooked	Turkey, all classes, (meat and skin, roasted)
Water (g)	40.20	12.32	55.49	60.60	59.45	60.70	30.52	49.78	61.70
Energy (Kcal)	458	541	278	247	239	201	466	339	208
Protein (g)	11.60	37.04	25.56	15.30	27.3	26.71	20.35	19.43	28.1
Total Fat (g)	45.04	41.78	18.74	19.87	13.6	9.63	40.28	28.36	9.73
Carbohy-drates (g)	0.66	1.43	0.0	0.73	0.0	0.0	4.04	0.0	0.0
Fiber (g)	0.0	0.0	0.0	0.0	0.0	0.0	1.5	0.0	0.0
Sugars, total (g)	0.0	0.0	0.0	0.0	0.0	0.0	0.75	0.0	0.0
Calcium (mg)	6	11	30	11	15	16	21	13	26
Iron (mg)	0.48	1.44	2.37	0.77	1.26	2.05	1.44	1.36	1.79
Magne-sium (mg)	12	33	20	14	23	24	18	17	25
Phospho-rus (mg)	188	533	189	139	182	207	176	163	203
Potassium (mg)	208	565	289	281	223	318	315	294	280
Sodium (mg)	833	2310	78	1184	82	80	1788	749	68
Zinc (mg)	1.17	3.50	6.19	2.03	1.94	5.14	2.73	2.08	2.96
Copper (mg)	0.07	0.164	0.075	0.080	0.066	0.153	0.071	0.086	0.093

MEAT	Bacon, raw	Bacon, broiled or fried	Beef, Ground, Broiled	Bologna, Pork	Chicken, meat & skin, roasted	Lamb	Pepperoni, pork, beef	Sausage, Pork, cooked	Turkey, all classes, (meat and skin, roasted)
Manganese (mg)	0.022	0.022	0.01	0.036	0.02	0.014	0.323	0.005	0.021
Selenium (mcg)	20.2	62.0	21.4	12.7	23.9	11.0	21.8	0.0	32.9
Vitamin C (mg)	0.0	0.0	0.0	0.0	0.0	0.0	0.7	0.7	0.0
Thiamin (mg)	0.281	0.404	0.049	0.523	0.063	0.131	0.532	0.294	0.057
Riboflavin (mg)	0.113	0.264	0.179	0.157	0.168	0.360	0.230	0.197	0.177
Niacin (mg)	3.828	11.099	4.818	3.90	8.487	5.812	5.416	6.258	5.086
Pantothenic acid (mg)	0.520	1.171	0.674	0.720	1.030	0.670	0.605	0.724	0.858
Vitamin B-6 (mg)	0.210	0.349	0.351	.270	0.4	0.394	0.39	0.327	0.410
Folate (mcg)	2	2	11	5	5	0.0	6	3	7
B-12 (mcg)	0.69	1.23	2.81	0.93	0.3	3.01	1.57	1.18	0.35
Vitamin A (IU)	37	37	0.0	0	157	0.0	0	79	0
Vitamin E (mg)	0.27	0.31	0.47	0.26	0.27	0.0	0.29	0.55	0.34
Vitamin D (IU)	0.0	0.0	0.0	56.0	0.0	0.0	9.419	0.0	0.0
Vitamin K (mcg)	0.0	0.1	2.1	0.3	2.4	0.0	1.3	0.4	0.9
Saturated Fat (g)	14.99	13.739	7.293	6.88	3.79	4.048	16.092	9.131	2.84
Cholesterol (mg)	68	110	89	59	88	87	118	84	82
Beta Carotene (mcg)	0.0	0.0	0.0	0.0	0	0.0	0	11	0
Alpha Carotene (mcg)	0.0	0.0	0.0	0.0	0	0.0	0	11	0

Values are per 100 grams of edible portion.

Some notes on the table: Bacon, sausage, and pepperoni are high in fat, in an approximate three to one ratio to protein. Some meats have more protein than fat, especially chicken and turkey, whose values above are for white and dark meat including the skin. There is minimal carbohydrate and no sugar in meat. There is no fiber. Meat contains some phosphorous, potassium, selenium and niacin. Most importantly, meat contains Vitamin B_{12}. Meat contains a small amount of calcium. Pork contains Vitamin D.

Dairy Products & Eggs	Milk, whole, 3.25% milk fat	Milk, 1% with Vitamin A	Milk, 1%, with	Yogurt, plain, low fat	Butter, unsalted	Ice cream, vanilla	Eggs	Egg yolk, 1 large
Water (g)	88.32	89.92	85.07	17.94	61.00	75.84	8.893
Energy (Kcal)	60	42	63	717	201	147	54.74
Protein (g)	3.22	3.37	5.25	0.85	3.50	12.58	2.696
Total Fat (g)	3.25	0.97	1.55	81.11	11.0	9.94	4.512
Carbohydrates (g)	4.52	4.99	7.04	0.06	23.6	0.77	0.610
Fiber (g)	0	0.0	0.0	0.0	0.7	0.0	0.0
Sugars, total (g)	5.26	5.2	7.04	0.06	21.22	0.77	0.095
Calcium (mg)	101	108	183	24	128	53	21.93
Iron (mg)	0.03	0.35	0.08	0.02	0.09	1.83	0.464
Magnesium (mg)	10	11	17	2	14	12	0.85
Phosphorus (mg)	84	89	144	24	105	191	66.3
Potassium (mg)	133	119	234	24	199	134	18.53
Sodium (mg)	43	50	70	11	80	140	8.16
Zinc (mg)	0.38	0.87	0.89	0.09	0.69	1.111	0.391
Copper (mg)	0.023	0.014	0.013	0.016	0.023	0.102	0.013
Manganese (mg)	0.003	0-035	0.004	0.004	0.008	0.038	0.009
Selenium (mcg)	3.7	3.3	3.3	1.0	1.8	31.7	9.52
Vitamin C (mg)	0.0	0.0	0.8	0.0	0.6	0.0	0.0
Thiamin (mg)	0.044	0.02	0.044	0.005	0.041	0.069	0.03

Dairy Products & Eggs	Milk, whole, 3.25% milk fat	Milk, 1%, with Vitamin A	Yogurt, plain, low fat	Butter, unsalted	Ice cream, vanilla	Eggs	Egg yolk, 1 large
Riboflavin (mg)	0.183	0.185	0.214	0.034	0.240	0.478	0.09
Niacin (mg)	0.107	0.093	0.114	0.042	0.116	0.070	0.004
Pantothenic acid (mg)	0.362	0.361	0.591	0.110	0.581	1.438	0.508
Vitamin B-6 (mg)	0.036	0.037	0.049	0.003	0.048	0.143	0.059
Folate (mcg)	5	5	11	3	5	47	24.82
B-12 (mcg)	0.44	0.44	0.56	0.17	0.39	1.29	0.331
Vitamin A (IU)	102	196	51	2499	422	487	245.14
Vitamin E (mg)	0.06	0.01	0.03	2.32	0.3	0.97	0.439
Vitamin D (IU)	40.43	51.95	0	0	34.73	34.54	18.26
Vitamin K (mcg)	0.2	0.1	0.2	7.0	0.3	0.3	0.119
Saturated Fat (g)	1.865	0.633	1.00	51.36	6.79	3.099	1.624
Cholesterol (mg)	10	5	6	215	44	423	209.78
Beta Carotene (mcg)	5	2	2	158	19	10	14.96
Alpha Carotene (mcg)	0	0	0	0	0	0	6.46

Note: Except for the egg yolk (last column), all values are for 100 grams of edible portion.

100 grams is equal to two large eggs or three small eggs.

The egg yolk values are for one large yolk.

Some notes on the table: Dairy products are rich in calcium. They are low in cholesterol and contain no fiber. Whole milk contains carbohydrate, protein, and fat in almost equal amounts. Milk contains phosphorous, magnesium, potassium, and small amounts of virtually every nutrient. Milk contains no Vitamin C and minimal Vitamin K and folate.

Our greatest source of Vitamin D is conversion from the inactive to the active metabolite caused by sunlight on our skin. We need twenty minutes of exposure daily to provide all our needs. Our second greatest source is fortified dairy products.

Ice cream has a similar profile to milk but contains more fat.

Butter is highest in total fat and saturated fat. Butter contains fewer nutrients across the board than milk except for large amounts of Vitamin A and moderately greater amounts of Vitamins E and K. All three of these, Vitamins A, E, and K, are fat soluble. Vitamin D, the fourth fat-soluble vitamin, is added to milk by the manufacturer and helps with the absorption of calcium needed for strong bones. Note that, when we consider butter, one hundred grams is a large portion but is used here for comparison. The healthiest diets avoid both butter and margarine. Some margarines now contain no trans fats and minimal saturated fat so they are healthier than before.

OILS	Canola	Coconut	Olive	Palm kernel	Peanut	Safflower	Soybean	Sunflower	Lard
Water (g)	0.0	0.0	0.0	0.0	0.0	0.0	0.0	0.0	0.0
Energy (Kcal)	123.76	117.23	119.34	117.23	119.34	120.22	120.22	123.76	115.45
Protein (g)	0.0	0.0	0.0	0.0	0.0	0.0	0.0	0.0	0.0
Total Fat (g)	14.0	13.6	13.5	13.6	13.5	13.6	13.6	14.0	12.8
Carbohydrates (g)	0.0	0.0	0.0	0.0	0.0	0.0	0.0	0.0	0.0
Fiber (g)	0.0	0.0	0.0	0.0	0.0	0.0	0.0	0.0	0.0
Sugars, total (g)	0.0	0.0	0.0	0.0	0.0	0.0	0.0	0.0	0.0
Calcium (mg)	0.0	0.0	0.135	0.0	0.0	0.0	0.0	0.0	0.0
Iron (mg)	0.0	0.005	0.089	0.0	0.004	0.0	0.003	0.0	0.0
Magnesium (mg)	0.0	0.0	0.0	0.0	0.0	0.0	0.0	0.0	0.0
Phosphorus (mg)	0.0	0.0	0.0	0.0	0.0	0.0	0.0	0.0	0.0
Potassium (mg)	0.0	0.0	0.135	0.0	0.0	0.0	0.0	0.0	0.0

OILS	Canola	Coconut	Olive	Palm kernel	Peanut	Safflower	Soybean	Sunflower	Lard
Sodium (mg)	0.0	0.0	0.405	0.0	0.0	0.0	0.0	0.0	0.0
Zinc (mg)	0.0	0.0	0.0	0.0	0.001	0.0	0.0	0.0	0.014
Copper (mg)	0.0	0.0	0.0	0.0	0.0	0.0	0.0	0.0	0.0
Manganese (mg)	0.0	0.0	0.0	0.0	0.0	0.0	0.0	0.0	0.0
Selenium (mcg)	0.0	0.0	0.0	0.0	0.0	0.0	0.0	0.0	0.026
Vitamin C (mg)	0.0	0.0	0.0	0.0	0.0	0.0	0.0	0.0	0.0
Thiamin (mg)	0.0	0.0	0.0	0.0	0.0	0.0	0.0	0.0	0.0
Riboflavin (mg)	0.0	0.0	0.0	0.0	0.0	0.0	0.0	0.0	0.0
Niacin (mg)	0.0	0.0	0.0	0.0	0.0	0.0	0.0	0.0	0.0
Pantothenic acid (mg)	0.0	0.0	0.0	0.0	0.0	0.0	0.0	0.0	0.0
Vitamin B-6 (mg)	0.0	0.0	0.0	0.0	0.0	0.0	0.0	0.0	0.0
Folate (mcg)	0.0	0.0	0.0	0.0	0.0	0.0	0.0	0.0	0.0
B-12 (mcg)	0.0	0.0	0.0	0.0	0.0	0.0	0.0	0.0	0.0
Vitamin A (IU)	0.0	0.0	0.0	0.0	0.0	0.0	0.0	0.0	0.0
Vitamin E (mg)	2.394	0.012	1.937	0.518	2.118	4.638	1.253	5.751	0.077
Vitamin K (mcg)	17.08	0.068	8.127	3.359	0.094	0.966	26.874	0.756	0.0
Saturated Fat (g)	0.994	11.764	1.816	11.084	2.281	0.844	1.958	1.365	5.018
Cholesterol (mg)	0.0	0.0	0.0	0.0	0.0	0.0	0.0	0.0	12.16

OILS	Canola	Coconut	Olive	Palm kernel	Peanut	Safflower	Soybean	Sunflower	Lard
Beta Carotene (mcg)	0.0	0.0	0.0	0.0	0.0	0.0	0.0	0.0	0.0
Alpha Carotene (mcg)	0.0	0.0	0.0	0.0	0.0	0.0	0.0	0.0	0.0

All values are per one tablespoon (about 13 – 14 grams, depending on how heavy the oil is).

Some thoughts on the table: Eight representative oils plus lard are profiled here. Oils derive all of their calories from fat. They contain no protein or carbohydrate, including no sugar. They contain no cholesterol. Most plant oils contain very little saturated fat. However, coconut and palm kernel oils each contain more than double the saturated fat of an equal amount of lard (palm oil contains slightly more saturated fat than lard, 6.7 grams to 5.01).

Most oils contain few nutrients. The oils derived from plants contain Vitamins E and K. The natural Vitamin E found in food may be more beneficial than Vitamin E found in supplements. Olive oil has a good reputation as an ingredient in the Mediterranean diet but doesn't stand out from the other oils in the nutrient table.

Olive, canola, and peanut oil contain monounsaturated fats. Monounsaturated oils may have protective effects on the heart and blood vessels and are considered the healthiest.

Corn, safflower, and fish oil contain polyunsaturated fats.

Lard, coconut, palm, and palm kernel oils contain saturated fats.

Any oils that the manufacturer alters, such as hydrogenated oils, also contain trans fat which is as harmful as saturated fat.

VEGETABLES TABLE 1	Artichokes	Asparagus	Avocado	Broccoli	Cabbage	Cauliflower	Carrots	Corn
Water (g)	84.94	93.22	73.23	89.30	92.15	91.91	88.29	75.96
Energy (Kcal)	47	20	160	34	24	25	41	86
Protein (g)	3.27	2.2	2.0	2.82	1.44	1.98	0.93	3.22
Total Fat (g)	0.15	0.12	14.6	0.37	0.12	0.10	0.24	1.18
Carbohydrates (g)	10.51	3.88	8.53	6.64	5.58	5.3	9.58	19.02
Fiber (g)	5.4	2.1	6.7	2.6	2.3	2.5	3.0	2.7
Sugars, total (g)	0	1.88	0.66	1.70	3.58	2.4	4.54	3.22
Calcium (mg)	44	24	12	47	47	22	33	2
Iron (mg)	1.28	2.14	0.55	0.73	0.59	0.44	0.30	0.52
Magnesium (mg)	60	14	29	21	15	15	12	37
Phosphorus (mg)	90	52	52	66	23	44	35	89
Potassium (mg)	370	202	485	316	246	303	320	270
Sodium (mg)	94	2	7	33	18	30	69	15
Zinc (mg)	0.49	0.54	0.64	0.41	0.18	0.28	0.24	0.45
Copper (mg)	0.23	0.18	0.19	0.049	0.023	0.042	0.045	0.054
Manganese (mg)	0.25	0.15	0.142	0.21	0.159	0.156	0.143	0.161
Selenium (mcg)	0.2	2.3	0.4	2.5	0.9	0.6	0.1	0.6
Vitamin C (mg)	11.7	5.6	10	89.2	32.2	46.4	5.9	6.8
Thiamin (mg)	0.07	0.143	0.067	0.071	0.05	0.057	0.066	0.2
Riboflavin (mg)	0.06	0.141	0.130	0.117	0.04	0.063	0.058	0.06
Niacin (mg)	1.04	0.978	1.738	0.639	0.30	0.526	0.983	1.7
Pantothenic acid (mg)	0.338	0.274	1.389	0.573	0.140	0.652	0.273	0.760
Vitamin B-6 (mg)	0.11	0.091	0.257	0.175	0.096	0.222	0.138	0.055
Folate (mcg)	68	52	58	63	43	57	19	46
B-12 (mcg)	0	0	0	0	0	0	0	0
Vitamin A (IU)	0	756	146	660	171	13	12036	208

VEGETABLES TABLE 1	Artichokes	Asparagus	Avocado	Broccoli	Cabbage	Cauliflower	Carrots	Corn
Vitamin E (mg)	0	1.13	2.07	0.78	0.15	0.08	0.66	0.07
Vitamin K (mcg)	14	41.6	21.0	101.6	60.0	16	13.2	0.3
Saturated Fat (g)	0.03	0.046	2.12	0.039	0.016	0.032	0.032	0.182
Cholesterol (mg)	0	0	0	0	0	0	0	0
Beta Carotene (mcg)	0	449	62	383	90	8	5774	52
Alpha Carotene (mcg)	0	9	24	25	25	0	2817	18

Values are for 100 grams of edible portion

VEGETABLES TABLE 2	Cucumber	Eggplant	Kale	Okra	Olives	Peas	Peppers, Green	Peppers, Red	Peppers, Yellow
Water (g)	95.23	92.41	84.46	90.17	79.99	78.86	93.89	92.21	92.02
Energy (Kcal)	15	24	50	31	115	81	20	26	27
Protein (g)	0.65	1.01	3.3	2.00	0.84	5.42	0.86	0.99	1.00
Total Fat (g)	0.11	0.19	0.7	0.1	10.68	0.4	0.17	0.3	0.21
Carbohydrates (g)	3.63	5.7	10.01	7.03	6.26	14.46	4.64	6.03	6.32
Fiber (g)	0.5	3.4	2.0	3.2	3.2	5.1	1.7	2.0	0.9
Sugars, total (g)	1.67	2.35	0	1.2	0	5.67	2.40	4.2	0
Calcium (mg)	16	9	135	81	88	25	10	7	11
Iron (mg)	0.28	0.24	1.7	0.8	3.3	1.47	0.34	0.43	0.46
Magnesium (mg)	13	14	34	57	4	33	10	12	12
Phosphorus (mg)	24	25	56	63	3	108	20	26	24
Potassium (mg)	147	230	447	303	8	244	175	211	212
Sodium (mg)	2	2	43	8	872	5	3	2	2
Zinc (mg)	0.2	0.016	0.44	0.6	0.22	1.24	0.13	0.25	0.17
Copper (mg)	0.041	0.082	0.29	0.094	0.251	0.176	0.066	0.017	0.107
Manganese (mg)	0.079	0.25	0.774	0.99	0.02	0.410	0.122	0.112	0.117
Selenium (mcg)	0.3	0.3	0.9	0.7	0.9	1.8	0	0.1	0.3
Vitamin C (mg)	2.8	2.2	120.0	21.1	0.9	40.0	80.4	190.0	183.5

VEGETABLES TABLE 2	Cucumber	Eggplant	Kale	Okra	Olives	Peas	Peppers, Green	Peppers, Red	Peppers, Yellow
Thiamin (mg)	0.027	0.039	0.11	0.2	0.003	0.266	0.057	0.054	0.028
Riboflavin (mg)	0.033	0.037	0.13	0.06	0.0	0.132	0.028	0.085	0.025
Niacin (mg)	0.098	0.649	1.0	1.0	0.037	2.09	0.480	0.979	0.89
Pantothenic acid (mg)	0.259	0.281	0.091	0.245	0.015	0.104	0.099	0.317	0.168
Vitamin B-6 (mg)	0.04	0.084	0.271	0.215	0.009	0.169	0.224	0.291	0.168
Folate (mcg)	7	22	29	88	0.0	65	11	18	26
B-12 (mcg)	0	0	0	0	0	0	0	0	0
Vitamin A (IU)	105	27	15376	375	403	765	370	3131	200
Vitamin E (mg)	0.03	0.3	0	0.36	1.65	0.13	0.37	1.58	0
Vitamin K (mcg)	16.4	3.5	817.0	53.0	1.4	24.8	7.4	4.9	0
Saturated Fat (g)	0.034	0.034	0.091	0.026	1.415	0.071	0.058	0.059	0.031
Cholesterol (mg)	0	0	0	0	0	0	0	0	0
Beta Carotene (mcg)	45	16	9226	225	237	449	208	1624	120
Alpha Carotene (mcg)	11	0	0	0	0	21	21	20	0

Values are for 100 grams of edible portion

VEGETABLES TABLE 3	Pumpkin	Spinach	Squash, Butter	Sweet potato	Swiss Chard	Tomatoes
Water (g)	91.60	91.40	86.41	79.78	92.66	94.50
Energy (Kcal)	26	23	45	76	19	18
Protein (g)	1.00	2.86	1.0	1.57	1.8	0.88
Total Fat (g)	0.10	0.39	0.1	0.05	0.2	0.2
Carbohydrates (g)	6.50	3.63	11.69	17.61	3.74	3.92
Fiber (g)	0.5	2.2	2.0	3.0	1.6	1.2
Sugars, total (g)	1.36	0.42	2.20	3.89	1.1	2.63
Calcium (mg)	21	99	48	30	51	10
Iron (mg)	0.8	2.71	0.70	0.61	1.8	0.27
Magnesium (mg)	12	79	34	25	81	11
Phosphorus (mg)	44	49	33	47	46	24
Potassium (mg)	340	558	352	337	379	237

VEGETABLES TABLE 3	Pumpkin	Spinach	Squash, Butter	Sweet potato	Swiss Chard	Tomatoes
Sodium (mg)	1	79	4	13	213	5
Zinc (mg)	0.32	0.53	0.15	0.3	0.36	0.17
Copper (mg)	0.127	0.13	0.072	0.151	0.179	0.059
Manganese (mg)	0.125	0.897	0.202	0.258	0.366	0.114
Selenium (mcg)	0.3	1.0	0.5	0.6	0.9	0
Vitamin C (mg)	9.0	28.1	21.0	22.7	30.0	12.7
Thiamin (mg)	0.05	0.078	0.1	0.078	0.04	0.037
Riboflavin (mg)	0.11	0.189	0.02	0.061	0.09	0.019
Niacin (mg)	0.6	0.724	1.2	0.557	0.4	0.594
Pantothenic acid	0.298	0.065	0.400	0.800	0.172	0.089
Vitamin B-6 (mg)	0.061	0.195	0.154	0.209	0.099	0.08
Folate (mcg)	16	194	27	14	14	15
B-12 (mcg)	0	0	0	0	0	0
Vitamin A (IU)	7384	9377	10630	14545	6116	833
Vitamin E (mg)	1.06	2.03	1.44	0.26	1.89	0.54
Vitamin K (mcg)	1.1	482.9	1.1	1.8	830.0	7.9
Saturated Fat (g)	0.052	0.063	0.021	0.018	0.03	0.045
Cholesterol (mg)	0	0	0	0	0	0
Beta Carotene (mcg)	3100	5626	4226	8727	3647	449
Alpha Carotene (mcg)	515	0	834	0	45	101

Values are for 100 grams of edible portion

Some thoughts on the tables: The calories in vegetables are mostly derived from carbohydrate. Generally, there is little sugar content, although carrots, corn, cabbage, and peas contain more sugar than most vegetables. Vegetables have minimal fat content, except for the avocado and olive, which still contain little compared to meat. There is no cholesterol. Vegetables do not contain any Vitamin B_{12} or Vitamin D. The government lists Vitamin B_{12} along the left hand column and then enters a "0" for each vegetable. The government does not list Vitamin D along the left hand column which also means zero content.

Vegetables contain small amounts of many nutrients, including

calcium, iron, magnesium, phosphorous, potassium, Vitamin C, niacin, and folate. Some nutrients vary widely from vegetable to vegetable. Carrots and spinach are high in Vitamin A; artichokes contain
no Vitamin A. As with fruits, an orange color usually means a hefty
dose of Vitamin A. Darker green vegetables like broccoli often contain Vitamin C, but red and yellow peppers contain more than twice
as much Vitamin C as green peppers.

Remember, deeply colored vegetables usually have more vitamins
and minerals than their lighter cousins. These include kale, spinach,
red pepper, and carrots. Many vegetables are rich sources of antioxidants. The best advice is to eat a wide variety of different vegetables.
Do not limit yourself to the same two or three vegetables every day.
Vary the colors.

FRUIT TABLE 1	Apples	Apricots	Bananas	Blackberries	Blueberries	Cantaloupe	Cherries	Grapefruit, pink
Water (g)	85.56	86.35	74.91	88.15	84.21	90.15	82.25	88.06
Energy (Kcal)	52	48	89	43	57	34	63	42
Protein (g)	0.26	1.40	1.09	1.39	0.74	0.84	1.06	0.77
Total Fat (g)	0.17	0.39	0.33	0.49	0.33	0.19	0.20	0.14
Carbohydrates (g)	13.81	11.12	22.84	9.61	14.49	8.16	16.01	10.66
Fiber (g)	2.4	2.0	2.6	5.3	2.4	0.9	2.1	1.6
Sugars, total (g)	10.39	9.24	12.23	4.88	9.96	7.86	12.82	6.89
Calcium (mg)	6	13	5	29	6	9	13	22
Iron (mg)	0.12	0.39	0.26	0.62	0.28	0.21	0.36	0.08
Magnesium (mg)	5	10	27	20	6	12	11	9
Phosphorus (mg)	11	23	22	22	12	15	21	18
Potassium (mg)	107	259	358	162	77	267	222	135
Sodium (mg)	1	1	1	1	1	16	0.0	0.0
Zinc (mg)	0.04	0.20	0.15	0.53	0.16	0.18	0.07	0.07
Copper (mg)	0.027	0.078	0.078	0.165	0.057	0.041	0.060	0.032

FRUIT TABLE 1	Apples	Apricots	Bananas	Blackberries	Blueberries	Cantaloupe	Cherries	Grapefruit, pink
Manganese (mg)	0.035	0.077	0.270	0.646	0.336	0.041	0.070	0.022
Selenium (mcg)	0.0	0.1	1.0	0.4	0.1	0.4	0.0	0.1
Vitamin C (mg)	4.6	10.0	8.7	21.0	9.7	36.7	7.0	31.2
Thiamin (mg)	0.017	0.03	0.031	0.02	0.037	0.041	0.027	0.043
Riboflavin (mg)	0.026	0.04	0.073	0.026	0.041	0.019	0.033	0.031
Niacin (mg)	0.091	0.60	0.665	0.646	0.418	0.734	0.154	0.204
Pantothenic acid	0.061	0.240	0.334	0.276	0.124	0.105	0.199	0.262
Vitamin B-6 (mg)	0.041	0.054	0.367	0.030	0.052	0.072	0.049	0.053
Folate (mcg)	3	9	20	25	6	21	4	13
B-12 (mcg)	0.0	0.0	0.0	0.0	0.0	0.0	0.0	0.0
Vitamin A (IU)	54	1926	64	214	54	3382	64	1150
Vitamin E (mg)	0.18	0.89	0.10	1.17	0.57	0.05	0.07	0.13
Vitamin K (mcg)	2.2	3.3	0.5	19.8	19.3	2.5	2.1	0.0
Saturated Fat (g)	0.028	0.027	0.112	0.014	0.028	0.051	0.038	0.020
Cholesterol (mg)	0.0	0.0	0.0	0.0	0.0	0.0	0.0	0.0
Beta Carotene (mcg)	27	1094	26	128	32	2020	38	686
Alpha Carotene (mcg)	0.0	19	25	0.0	0.0	16	0.0	3

Values are for 100 grams of edible portion.

FRUIT TABLE 2	Grapes	Guava	Honeydew	Kiwi	Mango	Oranges	Papaya	Peaches
Water (g)	81.30	86.10	89.82	83.07	81.71	86.75	88.83	88.87
Energy (Kcal)	67	51	36	61	65	47	39	39
Protein (g)	0.63	0.82	0.54	1.14	0.51	0.94	0.61	0.91
Total Fat (g)	0.35	0.60	0.14	0.52	0.27	0.12	0.14	0.25
Carbohydrates (g)	17.15	11.88	9.09	14.66	17.00	11.75	9.81	9.54

FRUIT TABLE 2	Grapes	Guava	Honeydew	Kiwi	Mango	Oranges	Papaya	Peaches
Fiber (g)	0.9	5.4	0.8	3.0	1.8	2.4	1.8	1.5
Sugars, total (g)	16.25	6.48	8.12	8.99	14.80	9.35	5.90	8.39
Calcium (mg)	14	20	6	34	10	40	24	6
Iron (mg)	0.29	0.31	0.17	0.31	0.13	0.10	0.10	0.25
Magnesium (mg)	5	10	10	17	9	10	10	9
Phosphorus (mg)	10	25	11	34	11	14	5	20
Potassium (mg)	191	284	228	312	156	181	257	190
Sodium (mg)	2	3	18	3	2	0	3	0.0
Zinc (mg)	0.04	0.23	0.09	0.14	0.04	0.07	0.07	0.17
Copper (mg)	0.04	0.103	0.024	0.130	0.11	0.045	0.016	0.068
Manganese (mg)	0.718	0.144	0.027	0.098	0.027	0.025	0.011	0.061
Selenium (mcg)	0.1	0.6	0.7	0.2	0.6	0.5	0.6	0.1
Vitamin C (mg)	4.0	183.5	18.0	92.7	27.7	53.2	61.8	6.6
Thiamin (mg)	0.092	0.05	0.038	0.027	0.058	0.087	0.027	0.024
Riboflavin (mg)	0.057	0.05	0.012	0.025	0.057	0.040	0.032	0.031
Niacin (mg)	0.30	1.2	0.418	0.341	0.584	0.282	0.338	0.806
Pantothenic acid (mg)	0.024	0.150	0.155	0.183	0.160	0.250	0.218	0.153
Vitamin B-6 (mg)	0.11	0.143	0.088	0.063	0.134	0.060	0.019	0.025
Folate (mcg)	4	14	19	25	14	30	38	4
B-12 (mcg)	0.0	0.0	0.0	0.0	0.0	0.0	0.0	0.0
Vitamin A (IU)	100	624	50	87	765	225	1094	326
Vitamin E (mg)	0.19	0.73	0.02	1.46	1.12	0.18	0.73	0.73
Vitamin K (mcg)	14.6	2.6	2.9	40.3	4.2	0.0	2.6	2.6
Saturated Fat (g)	0.114	0.172	0.038	0.029	0.066	0.015	0.043	0.019
Cholesterol (mg)	0.0	0.0	0.0	0.0	0.0	0.0	0.0	0.0
Beta Carotene (mcg)	59	374	30	52	445	71	276	162
Alpha Carotene (mcg)	1	0.0	0.0	0.0	17	11	0.0	0.0

Values are for 100 grams of edible portion

FRUIT TABLE 3	Pineapple	Plums	Raspberries	Rhubarb	Strawberries	Watermelon
Water (g)	86.46	87.23	85.75	93.61	90.95	91.45
Energy (Kcal)	48	46	52	21	32	30
Protein (g)	0.54	0.70	1.20	0.90	0.67	0.61
Total Fat (g)	0.12	0.28	0.65	0.20	0.3	0.15
Carbohydrates (g)	12.63	11.42	11.94	4.54	7.68	7.55
Fiber (g)	1.4	1.4	6.5	1.8	2.0	0.4
Sugars, total (g)	9.26	9.92	4.42	1.1	4.66	6.2
Calcium (mg)	13	6	25	86	16	7
Iron (mg)	0.28	0.17	0.69	0.22	0.42	0.24
Magnesium (mg)	12	7	22	12	13	10
Phosphorus (mg)	8	16	29	14	24	11
Potassium (mg)	115	157	151	288	153	112
Sodium (mg)	1	0.0	1	4	1	1
Zinc (mg)	0.1	0.1	0.42	0.1	0.14	0.10
Copper (mg)	0.099	0.057	0.09	0.021	0.048	0.042
Manganese (mg)	1.177	0.052	0.67	0.196	0.386	0.038
Selenium (mcg)	0.1	0.0	0.2	1.1	0.4	0.4
Vitamin C (mg)	36.2	9.5	26.2	8.0	58.8	8.1
Thiamin (mg)	0.079	0.028	0.032	0.02	0.024	0.033
Riboflavin (mg)	0.031	0.026	0.038	0.03	0.022	0.021
Niacin (mg)	0.489	0.417	0.598	0.30	0.386	0.178
Pantothenic acid (mg)	0.205	0.135	0.329	0.085	0.125	0.221
Vitamin B-6 (mg)	0.110	0.029	0.055	0.024	0.047	0.045
Folate (mcg)	15	5	21	7	24	3
B-12 (mcg)	0.0	0.0	0.0	0.0	0.0	0.0
Vitamin A (IU)	56	345	33	102	12	569
Vitamin E (mg)	0.02	0.26	0.87	0.38	0.29	0.05
Vitamin K (mcg)	0.7	6.4	7.8	41	2.2	0.1
Saturated Fat (g)	0.009	0.017	0.019	0.053	0.015	0.016
Cholesterol (mg)	0.0	0.0	0.0	0.0	0.0	0.0
Beta Carotene (mcg)	34	190	12	61	7	303
Alpha Carotene (mcg)	0.0	0.0	16	0.0	0.0	0.0

Values are for 100 grams of edible portion

Some thoughts on the tables: Fruits contain no cholesterol and only a tiny amount of saturated fat. They contain minimal protein. They are high in carbohydrates, one-half to two-thirds of which are sugars. Again, this varies among the individual fruits. Grapes contain fifteen times as much total sugar as rhubarb, 16.2 grams compared to 1.1 grams. Apples, bananas, cherries, and mangoes all contain more than ten grams of sugar per one hundred grams of edible fruit. Diabetics in particular must be cautious with fruit intake, especially those fruits highest in sugar content.

Fruits are rich in fiber. Blackberries, guava, and raspberries all contain more than five grams of fiber per one hundred gram serving.

Fruits are a good source of Vitamin A, Vitamin C, and potassium. The orange fruits in particular, such as apricots, cantaloupe, mango, and peaches, contain a significant amount of Vitamin A, but so do plums and watermelon. Fruits contain minimal iron. They contain no Vitamin B_{12} or Vitamin D. Many fruits are rich sources of antioxidants.

FRUIT JUICES	Apple, canned or bottled	Cranberry, unsweetened	Grape, canned or bottled	Grapefruit, pink, raw	Orange, raw	Pineapple, canned, unsweetened	Prune, canned	Tomato, canned, without added salt
Water (g)	87.93	87.13	84.12	90.0	88.30	85.53	81.24	93.9
Energy (Kcal)	47	46	61	39	45	56	71	17
Protein (g)	0.06	0.39	0.56	0.5	0.70	0.32	0.61	0.76
Total Fat (g)	0.11	0.13	0.08	0.10	0.20	0.08	0.03	0.05
Carbohydrates (g)	11.68	12.20	14.96	9.20	10.40	13.78	17.45	4.24
Fiber (g)	0.1	0.1	0.1	NA	0.2	0.2	1.0	0.4
Sugars, total (g)	10.90	12.10	14.86	NA	8.40	13.58	16.45	3.56
Calcium (mg)	7	8	9	9	11	17	12	10
Iron (mg)	0.37	0.25	0.24	0.2	0.20	0.26	1.18	0.43
Magnesium (mg)	3	6	10	12	11	13	14	11
Phosphorus (mg)	7	13	11	15	17	8	25	18
Potassium (mg)	119	77	132	162	200	134	276	229
Sodium (mg)	3	2	3	1	1	1	4	10
Zinc (mg)	0.3	0.1	0.05	0.05	0.05	0.11	0.21	0.15
Copper (mg)	0.022	0.055	0.028	0.033	0.044	0.09	0.068	0.061
Manganese (mg)	0.113	0	0.360	0.020	0.014	0.990	0.151	0.07
Selenium (mcg)	0.1	0.1	0.1	0.0	0.1	0.1	0.6	0.3

FRUIT JUICES	Apple, canned or bottled	Cranberry, unsweetened	Grape, canned or bottled	Grapefruit, pink, raw	Orange, raw	Pineapple, canned, unsweetened	Prune, canned	Tomato, canned, without added salt
Vitamin C (mg)	0.9	9.3	0.1	38.0	50.0	10.7	4.1	18.3
Thiamin (mg)	0.021	0.009	0.026	0.04	0.09	0.055	0.016	0.047
Riboflavin (mg)	0.017	0.018	0.037	0.02	0.030	0.022	0.070	0.031
Niacin (mg)	0.1	0.091	0.262	0.20	0.400	0.257	0.785	0.673
Pantothenic acid (mg)	0.063	0	0.041	0.189	0.19	0.10	0.107	0.250
Vitamin B-6 (mg)	0.03	0.052	0.065	0.044	0.040	0.096	0.218	0.111
Folate (mcg)	0	1	3	10	30	23	0	20
B-12 (mcg)	0	0	0.0	0.00	0.0	0.0	0.0	0.0
Vitamin A (IU)	1	45	8	440	200	5	3	450
Vitamin E (mg)	0.01	1.2	0.0	0	0.04	0.02	0.12	0.32
Vitamin K (mcg)	0	5.1	0.4	0	0.1	0.3	3.4	2.3
Saturated Fat (g)	0.019	0.01	0.025	0.014	0.024	0.005	0.003	0.008
Cholesterol (mg)	0	0	0	0	0	0	0	0
Beta Carotene (mcg)	0	27	5	0	33	3	2	270
Alpha Carotene (mcg)	0	0	0	0	6	0	0	0

Values are for 100 grams of edible portion

Note: These values are for unsweetened juice without added salt. The orange and grapefruit juice values are for the raw juices; the other values are for canned juices

A few thoughts on the table: Juices contain a modest amount of calories, from a low of seventeen for tomato to a high of seventy-one for prune juice. They contain virtually no fat or protein, only carbohydrates, almost all of which are sugars. Diabetics need to exercise caution. Tomato juice is by far the lowest in sugar, which may be one reason people tend to think of the tomato as a vegetable rather than a fruit However, the tomato is a fruit.

Fruit juices are a great source of potassium, helpful to those who need extra amounts of this electrolyte in their diet, such as patients taking a diuretic, the medical name for a "water pill" that increases urine output. Unless salt is added, fruit juices are extremely low in sodium. All contain modest amounts of calcium and phosphorous, plus small amounts of many other vitamins and minerals.

A few nutrients are lost in going from the fruit to the juice. For example, if we compare the tables, apple juice contains less fiber, Vitamin C, and folate than the fruit itself; orange juice contains less fiber, calcium, and selenium than the fruit. Interestingly, the grams of water changes relatively little. All fruits and fruit juices are 80 to 95% water, with one exception - the banana, which is only 75% water. So, both the fruit and fruit juices are excellent means to replace lost body fluids.

BEANS	Black	Garbanzo, Chickpeas	Kidney	Lentils	Navy	Pinto	Soy	White
Water (g)	11.02	11.53	11.75	11.19	12.36	16.54	67.5	11.32
Energy (Kcal)	341	364	333	338	335	318	147	333
Protein (g)	21.6	19.3	23.58	28.06	22.33	20.70	12.95	23.36
Total Fat (g)	1.42	6.04	0.83	0.96	1.28	1.35	6.80	0.85
Carbohydrates (g)	62.36	60.65	60.01	57.09	60.66	57.75	11.05	60.27
Fiber (g)	15.2	17.4	24.9	30.5	24.4	15.5	4.2	15.2
Sugars, total (g)	2.25	10.70	2.23	5.40	2.22	2.11	0	2.24
Calcium (mg)	123	105	143	51	155	107	197	240
Iron (mg)	5.02	6.24	8.2	9.02	6.44	5.15	3.55	10.44
Magnesium (mg)	171	115	140	1.429	173	176	65	190
Phosphorus (mg)	352	366	407	454	443	401	194	301
Potassium (mg)	1483	875	1406	905	1140	1413	620	1795
Sodium (mg)	5	24	24	10	14	17	15	16
Zinc (mg)	3.65	3.43	2.79	3.61	2.54	2.56	0.99	3.67
Copper (mg)	0.841	0.847	0.958	0.852	0.879	0.788	0.128	0.984
Manganese (mg)	1.06	2.204	1.021	1.429	1.309	1.167	0.547	1.796
Selenium (mcg)	3.2	8.2	3.2	8.2	11.0	27.9	1.5	12.8
Vitamin C (mg)	0.0	4.0	4.5	6.2	3.0	6.3	29.0	0
Thiamin (mg)	0.90	0.477	0.529	0.475	0.645	0.512	0.435	0.437
Riboflavin (mg)	0.193	0.212	0.219	0.245	0.232	0.339	0.175	0.146
Niacin (mg)	1.955	1.541	2.060	2.621	2.063	1.447	1.65	0.479

BEANS	Black	Garbanzo, Chickpeas	Kidney	Lentils	Navy	Pinto	Soy	White
Pantothenic acid (mg)	0.899	1.588	0.780	1.849	0.680	0.485	0.147	0.732
Vitamin B-6 (mg)	0.286	0.535	0.397	0.535	0.437	0.553	0.065	0.318
Folate (mcg)	444	557	394	433	370	506	165	388
B-12 (mcg)	0.0	0	0.0	0.0	0	0.00	0	0
Vitamin A (IU)	0	67	0.0	39	0	0	0	0
Vitamin E (mg)	0.22	0.82	0.22	0.33	0.34	0.21	0	0.22
Vitamin K (mcg)	6.0	9.0	19.0	5.0	2.0	5.6	0	5.9
Saturated Fat (g)	0.366	0.626	0.12	0.135	0.331	0.235	0.786	0.219
Cholesterol (mg)	0	0	0	0	0	0	0	0
Beta Carotene (mcg)	0	40	0	23	0	0	0	0
Alpha Carotene (mcg)	0	0	0	0	0	0	0	0

Values are per 100 grams of edible portion.

Some thoughts on the table: Beans are a good source of carbo-hydrate and protein. They contain little fat, except for garbanzo and soy beans, which contain modest amounts of unsaturated fat. Beans contain no cholesterol. They are an excellent source of fiber, except for soybeans, which contain a more modest amount.

Beans are a fantastic source of many nutrients, including iron, magnesium, phosphorous, potassium, zinc, manganese, selenium, and niacin. Some contain small amounts of Vitamins A and K. Like fruits, vegetables, oils, and nuts, they contain no Vitamin B_{12} or Vitamin D.

GRAINS	Barley	Bulgur	Millet	Oats	Quinoa	Rice, Brown	Wheat flour, Whole grain	Wheat germ	Wheat flour, White, unenriched
Water (g)	9.44	9.00	8.67	8.22	9.30	10.37	10.27	11.12	11.92
Energy (Kcal)	354	342	378	389	374	370	339	360	364
Protein (g)	12.48	12.29	11.02	16.89	13.10	7.94	13.7	23.15	10.33
Total Fat (g)	2.30	1.33	4.22	6.90	5.80	2.92	1.87	9.72	0.98
Carbohy-drates (g)	73.48	75.87	72.85	66.27	68.9	77.24	72.57	51.8	76.31
Fiber (g)	17.3	18.3	8.5	10.6	5.9	3.5	12.2	13.2	2.7
Sugars, total (g)	0.80	0.41	0.0	0.0	0.0	0.85	0.41	0.0	0.27
Calcium (mg)	33	35	8	54	60	23	34	39	15
Iron (mg)	3.60	2.46	3.01	4.72	9.25	1.47	3.88	6.26	1.17
Magnesium (mg)	133	164	114	177	210	143	138	239	22
Phosphorus (mg)	264	300	285	523	410	333	346	842	108
Potassium (mg)	452	410	195	429	740	223	405	892	107
Sodium (mg)	12	17	5	2	21	7	5	12	2
Zinc (mg)	2.77	1.93	1.68	3.97	3.3	2.02	2.93	12.29	0.70
Copper (mg)	0.498	0.335	0.75	0.626	0.82	0.277	0.382	0.796	0.144
Manganese (mg)	1.943	3.038	1.632	4.916	2.26	3.743	3.799	13.30	0.682
Selenium (mcg)	37.7	2.3	2.7	0.0	0.0	23.4	70.7	79.2	33.9
Vitamin C (mg)	0.0	0.0	0.0	0.0	0.0	0.0	0.0	0.0	0.0
Thiamin (mg)	0.646	0.232	0.421	0.763	0.198	0.401	0.447	1.882	0.12
Riboflavin (mg)	0.285	0.115	0.290	0.139	0.396	0.093	0.215	0.499	0.04
Niacin (mg)	4.604	5.114	4.72	0.961	2.93	5.091	6.365	6.813	1.25

GRAINS	Barley	Bulgur	Millet	Oats	Quinoa	Rice, Brown	Wheat flour, Whole grain	Wheat germ	Wheat flour, White, unenriched
Pantothenic acid (mg)	0.282	1.045	0.848	1.349	1.047	1.493	1.008	2.257	0.438
Vitamin B-6 (mg)	0.318	0.342	0.384	0.119	0.223	0.509	0.341	1.3	0.044
Folate (mcg)	19	27	85	56	49	20	44	281	26
B-12 (mcg)	0.0	0.0	0.0	0.0	0.0	0.0	0.0	0.0	0.0
Vitamin A (IU)	22	9	0.0	0.0	0.0	0.0	9	0.0	0.0
Vitamin E (mg)	0.57	0.06	0.05	0.0	0.0	1.2	0.82	0.0	0.06
Vitamin K (mcg)	2.2	1.9	0.9	0.0	0.0	1.9	1.9	0.0	0.3
Saturated Fat (g)	0.482	0.232	0.723	1.217	0.59	0.584	0.322	1.665	0.155
Cholesterol (mg)	0.0	0.0	0.0	0.0	0.0	0.0	0.0	0.0	0.0
Beta Caro-tene (mcg)	13	5	0.0	0.0	0.0	0.0	5	0.0	0.0
Alpha Caro-tene (mcg)	0.0	0.0	0.0	0.0	0.0	0.0	0	0.0	0.0

Values are for 100 grams of edible portion.

Some thoughts on the table: Grains are a good source of protein and carbohydrate, very little of which is sugar. Grains are low in fat, especially saturated fat. They contain no cholesterol.

Grains are a good source of many nutrients, including iron, magnesium, phosphorous, potassium, zinc, manganese, selenium, and niacin. They contain modest amounts of calcium. Some have a small amount of Vitamins A and K.

Like fruits, vegetables, oils, nuts, and beans, they contain no Vitamin B$_{12}$ or Vitamin D. Nature may have grown accustomed to humans who ate meat and got sunlight.

SEAFOOD TABLE 1	Catfish	Cod, Atlantic	Flounder	Haddock	Halibut	Herring, Atlantic	Lobster
Water (g)	80.36	81.22	79.06	79.92	77.92	72.05	76.76
Energy (Kcal)	95	82	91	87	110	158	90
Protein (g)	16.38	17.81	18.84	18.91	20.81	17.96	18.80
Total Fat (g)	2.82	0.67	1.19	0.72	2.29	9.04	0.90
Carbohydrates (g)	0.00	0.00	0.0	0.0	0.0	0.0	0.50
Fiber (g)	0.00	0.00	0.0	0.0	0.0	0.0	0.0
Sugars, total (g)	0.00	0.00	0.0	0.0	0.0	0.0	0.0
Calcium (mg)	14	16	18	33	47	57	48
Iron (mg)	0.30	0.38	0.36	1.05	0.84	1.10	0.30
Magnesium (mg)	23	32	31	39	83	32	27
Phosphorus (mg)	209	203	184	188	222	236	144
Potassium (mg)	358	413	361	311	450	327	275
Sodium (mg)	43	54	81	68	54	90	296
Zinc (mg)	0.51	0.45	0.45	0.37	0.42	0.99	3.02
Copper (mg)	0.034	0.028	0.32	0.026	0.027	0.092	1.663
Manganese (mg)	0.025	0.015	0.017	0.025	0.015	0.035	0.055
Selenium (mcg)	12.6	33.1	32.7	30.2	36.5	36.5	41.4
Vitamin C (mg)	0.7	1.0	1.7	0.0	0.0	0.7	0.0
Thiamin (mg)	0.210	0.076	0.089	0.035	0.06	0.092	0.006
Riboflavin (mg)	0.072	0.065	0.076	0.037	0.075	0.233	0.048
Niacin (mg)	1.907	2.063	2.899	3.803	5.848	3.217	1.455
Pantothenic acid (mg)	0.765	0.153	0.503	0.127	0.329	0.645	1.630
Vitamin B-6 (mg)	0.116	0.245	0.208	0.30	0.344	0.302	0.063
Folate (mcg)	10	7	8	12	12	10	9
B-12 (mcg)	2.23	0.91	1.52	1.2	1.18	13.67	0.93
Vitamin A (IU)	50	12	33	57	157	93	70
Vitamin E (mg)	0	0.64	0.51	0.39	0.85	1.07	1.47
Vitamin D (IU)	500.0	44.0	60.0	0.0	0.0	1628	0.0
Vitamin K (mcg)	0	0.1	0.1	0.1	0.1	0.1	0.1
Saturated Fat (g)	0.722	0.131	0.283	0.130	0.325	2.04	0.180
Cholesterol (mg)	58	43	48	57	32	60	95
Beta Carotene (mcg)	0	0	0	0	0	0	0
Alpha Carotene (mcg)	0	0	0	0	0	0	0

All values are per 100 grams of edible portion, raw.

SEAFOOD TABLE 2	Oyster, Pacific	Salmon, Atlantic	Sardines, Atlantic, canned in oil	Sardines, Pacific, canned in tomato sauce	Shrimp	Trout	Tuna, canned in water
Water (g)	82.06	68.50	59.61	66.65	75.86	71.87	75.21
Energy (Kcal)	81	142	208	186	106	119	116
Protein (g)	9.45	19.84	24.62	20.86	20.31	20.48	25.51
Total Fat (g)	2.30	6.34	11.45	10.46	1.73	3.46	0.82
Carbohydrates (g)	4.95	0.0	0.0	0.74	0.91	0.0	0.0
Fiber (g)	0.0	0.0	0.0	0.1	0.0	0.0	0.0
Sugars, total (g)	0.0	0.0	0.0	0.43	0.0	0.0	0.0
Calcium (mg)	8	12	382	240	52	67	11
Iron (mg)	5.11	0.80	2.92	2.30	2.41	0.70	1.53
Magnesium (mg)	22	29	39	34	37	31	27
Phosphorus (mg)	162	200	490	366	205	271	163
Potassium (mg)	168	490	397	341	185	481	237
Sodium (mg)	106	44	505	414	148	31	50
Zinc (mg)	16.62	0.64	1.31	1.40	1.11	1.08	0.077
Copper (mg)	1.576	0.250	0.186	0.272	0.264	0.109	0.051
Manganese (mg)	0.643	0.016	0.108	0.206	0.050	0.158	0.011
Selenium (mcg)	77.0	36.5	52.7	40.6	38.0	12.6	80.4
Vitamin C (mg)	8.0	0.0	0.0	1.0	2.0	2.4	0.0
Thiamin (mg)	0.067	0.226	0.080	0.044	0.028	0.123	0.032
Riboflavin (mg)	0.233	0.380	0.227	0.233	0.034	0.105	0.074
Niacin (mg)	2.010	7.86	5.245	4.2	2.552	5.384	13.28
Pantothenic acid (mg)	0.500	1.664	0.642	0.730	0.276	0.928	0.214
Vitamin B-6 (mg)	0.050	0.818	0.167	0.123	0.104	0.406	0.350
Folate (mcg)	10	25	12	24	3	12	4
B-12 (mcg)	16.0	3.18	8.94	9.0	1.16	4.45	2.99
Vitamin A (IU)	270	12	108	143	180	62	56
Vitamin E (mg)	0.0	0.0	2.04	1.44	1.10	0.0	0.0
Vitamin D (IU)	0.0	0.0	272.0	480	152.0	0.0	0.0
Vitamin K (mcg)	0.0	0.0	2.6	0.4	0.0	0.0	0.0
Saturated Fat (g)	0.510	0.981	1.528	2.686	0.328	0.722	0.234
Cholesterol (mg)	50	55	142	61	152	59	30
Beta Carotene (mcg)	0.0	0.0	0.0	21	0.0	0.0	0.0
Alpha Carotene (mcg)	0.0	0.0	0.0	0.0	0.0	0.0	0.0

All values are per 100 grams of edible portion.

Some thoughts on the tables: Seafood is a great source of protein. Most seafood contains no carbohydrate, except for oysters. Seafood is low in fat, except for certain species, such as herring and sardines, both of which are rare in that they contain both significant amounts of natural calcium and Vitamin D, a great combination. Catfish, cod, flounder, and shrimp also contain both calcium and Vitamin D but in lesser amounts. Very few foods contain both calcium and Vitamin D unless they are fortified.

Patients who don't drink milk or get sunlight should consume these fish frequently. Seafood is low in cholesterol and contains no fiber.

Fish are a good source of Vitamin B_{12}, especially herring and oysters. Oysters are also rich in zinc which may be the reason that some advocates endow them with aphrodisiac qualities.

Appendix D - Healthy Hannah and Fat Freddy

This comparison will help those who want to be their own nutritionist or who need to keep close track of how much they consume of any particular nutrient or ingredient, including calories, sodium, saturated fat, and sugar. As such, it may contain more information than most readers need.

Let's take a look at the breakfast of two hypothetical people whom we'll call Healthy Hannah and Fat Freddy. Hannah watches her diet carefully and eats balanced, healthy meals. Freddy eats what he likes.

Here is Hannah's breakfast. Unless otherwise noted, assume that all portions are 100 grams (3.5 ounces):

Breakfast
Shredded wheat cereal
Low fat 1% milk, 200 grams
One large banana

Now, let's break down the nutrient value of her meal. Most of these numbers are found in the tables Appendix C. You'll find some of them on the nutrition label of the food, for example, the doughnuts. We'll look at the following items:

Energy (Kilocalories)   Total fat (grams)
Protein (grams)   Carbohydrates (grams)

Fiber (grams)
Total sugars (grams)
Calcium (milligrams)
Iron (milligrams)
Sodium (milligrams)

Vitamin C (milligrams)
Vitamin B12 (micrograms)
Saturated fatty acids (grams)
Cholesterol (milligrams)

HEALTHY BREAKFAST	Shredded Wheat Cereal	Banana	1% Milk	Totals
Energy (Kcal)	340	89	42	471
Protein (g)	10.40	1.09	3.37	14.86
Total fat (g)	1.20	0.33	0.97	2.5
Carbohydrates (g)	82.90	22.84	4.99	110.73
Fiber (g)	11.5	2.6	0	14.1
Sugars (g)	0.80	12.23	5.20	18.23
Calcium (mg)	44	5	108	157
Iron (mg)	3.13	0.26	0.35	3.74
Sodium (mg)	7	1	50	58
Vitamin C (mg)	0	8.7	0	8.7
Vitamin B-12 (mcg)	0	0	0.44	0
Fatty acids, total saturated (g)	0.2	0.112	0.633	0.945
Cholesterol (mg)	0	0	5	5

Here's Fred's breakfast:

Breakfast
Two large eggs
Bacon
Two chocolate donuts (cake style)
Two glasses whole milk (3.25% milk fat)

Now, let's look at a similar table:

UNHEALTHY BREAKFAST	Two large eggs	Bacon	Two Chocolate Donuts	100 g whole milk	Totals
Energy (Kcal)	147	541	417	60	1165
Protein (g)	12.58	37.04	4.5	3.22	57.34
Total fat (g)	9.94	41.78	19.9	3.25	74.87
Carbohydrates (g)	0.77	1.43	57.4	4.52	64.12
Fiber (g)	0	0	2.2	0	2.2
Sugars (g)	0.77	0	31.92	5.26	37.95
Calcium (mg)	53	11	213	101	378
Iron (mg)	1.83	1.44	2.27	0.03	5.57
Sodium (mg)	140	2310	340	43	2833
Vitamin C (mg)	0	0	0.1	0	0.1
Vitamin B-12 (mcg)	1.29	1.23	0.1	0.44	3.06
Fatty acids, total saturated (g)	3.099	13.739	5.132	1.865	23.835
Cholesterol	423	110	57	10	600

A COMPARISON

Now, we can put the meals side by side and see where the differences lie. Here is a comparison table:

COMPARISON, INDIVIDUAL MEALS	Healthy Breakfast	Unhealthy Breakfast
Energy (Kcal)	471	1165
Protein (g)	14.86	57.34
Total fat (g)	2.5	74.87
Carbohydrates (g)	110.73	64.12
Fiber (g)	14.1	2.2
Sugars (g)	18.23	37.95
Calcium (mg)	157	378
Iron (mg)	3.74	5.57
Sodium (mg)	58	2833
Vitamin C (mg)	8.7	0.1
Vitamin B-12 (mcg)	0	3.06
Fatty acids, total saturated (g)	0.945	23.835
Cholesterol	5	600

Here's how the two compare when we break down the components of their meal:

Calories: Freddy consumed twice as many calories as Hannah.

Fat: Freddy consumed thirty times as much fat as Hannah.

Fiber: Hannah consumed over six times as much fiber as Freddy.

Sodium: Freddy consumed about fifty times as much sodium as Hannah.

Cholesterol: Fat Freddy consumed a whopping one hundred twenty times as much cholesterol as Hannah.

Note that Freddy did get more calcium and iron than Hannah. Also, Hannah consumed no Vitamin B_{12} from her meat-free breakfast. Remember that more restricted diets can lack essential nutrients. Hannah can make up the differences later in the day.

From this comparison, we can see what a tremendous difference one meal makes. Now, consider the effects of this diet after three meals a day, 365 days a year, for a lifetime.

Start your new, powerful day with a great breakfast.

Index

Author Biography

Michael Grusenmeyer, M.D., has practiced medicine as a family doctor and emergency physician for 30 years. He graduated from the University of Michigan in Ann Arbor with a B.S. in Zoology and Chemistry. He obtained his medical degree from Wayne State University in Detroit. He is licensed in five states: Ohio, Michigan, Arizona, North Carolina, and California. He has worked as a consultant to the Cleveland Clinic Foundation, University Hospitals of Cleveland, the United States Navy, and the United States Air Force. He currently resides in Rocky River, Ohio.

www.ingramcontent.com/pod-product-compliance
Lightning Source LLC
Chambersburg PA
CBHW062143280526
45788CB00001B/279